Dr. Jane's
30 Days to a Healthier,
Happier Cat

Dr. Jane's 30 Days to a Healthier, Happier Cat

Jane R. Bicks, D.V.M.

Illustrations by Ouida McIlhinney

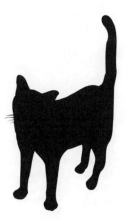

A Perigee Book

A Perigee Book
Published by The Berkley Publishing Group
200 Madison Avenue
New York, NY 10016

Perigee Special Sales edition: December 1996
ISBN: 0-399-52317-0

Published simultaneously in Canada.

The Putnam Berkley World Wide Web site address is
http://www.berkley.com/berkley

This book is not intended as a substitute for the medical
advice of a doctor of veterinary medicine. The reader should
regularly consult a veterinarian in matters relating to his pet's
health and particularly with respect to any symptoms that may
require diagnosis or medical attention.

Printed in the United States of America

10   9   8   7   6   5   4   3   2   1

Contents

. . . .

Part One
Feeding to Win

Part Two
Feeding the Right Stuff

Part Three
Getting Better All the Time

Part Four
Dr. Jane's New-Life Nutrition Plan

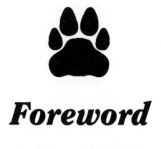

Foreword

Somewhere between forty-five and fifty-five centuries ago, in Egypt, man in his wisdom took the cat into his home, his life, and his heart.

Very shortly after the cat's descent into domestication it was elevated to godhood, and Basht emerged as a goddess for whom many strange forms of propitiation were required. It became a crime punishable by death to kill a cat. If a cat died, the family was expected to shave their heads, rub ashes over themselves, slash their clothes, and go around for specified periods of time in deep mourning. Cats, when they died, were mummified just as upper class human beings were, and a cemetery was established in a city called Bastet, named after the cat goddess, where hundreds of thousands of mummified cats were interred.

Eventually the cat was carried from North Africa and the Middle East to Europe, where the cat became, instead of a goddess, the familiar of devils and witches. Legend has it that Queen Elizabeth, in a somewhat over-played religious fervor, had a life-size straw model of the Pope made and filled with live cats. Then she is said to have personally set the figure on fire so that the screams of the burning cats would express her feelings about the Roman church. It was a long way from godhood to helpless sacrifice to religious bigotry.

For all of its ups and downs, the cat has stayed with us as a beloved companion to this very day. It has been treated with various degrees of awe, deep and profound love, and unfortunately, with disdain and neglect. Life is a very mixed bag of tricks for a kitten facing cathood.

Dr. Jane R. Bicks, a veterinarian who serves her patients with love as well as medical wisdom, has written *30 Days to a Healthier, Happier Cat*. It matters very much to Dr. Jane to have as many cats as possible be as happy as possible, and she can guide the owner toward these goals.

For all of their intelligence, cats really cannot handle the complexities of the modern world. The way they are forced to live they seldom can obtain the nutrition they need, and are crowded into living accommodations designed for us and not for them. They are frequently exposed to communicable diseases.

It is true that cats are extraordinarily manipulative animals, but what they can manipulate is their human companions, not the world they share with people. Nutrition is of extreme importance, as is the early identification of problems. Anyone who considers himself a cat lover and a cat owner is morally, ethically, and intellectually responsible for making sure the cat gets the nutritionally balanced diet it needs.

Anyone taking Jane R. Bicks's book in hand—paying careful heed to the matters she addresses so well—will have taken one giant step in the direction of responsible pet ownership and true cat loving. It's a book I commend to all my fellow feline enthusiasts without qualification or restraint.

Roger A. Caras
Thistle Hill Farm

Acknowledgments

• •

This book is lovingly dedicated to all the thousands of animal owners, veterinarians, and other animal health workers that have sought to prevent and or cure problems in pets using a holistic approach. If it were not for my husband, James Rapp, there would not have been a book. He supported my continuous effort to study herbal and nutritional medicine, and provided me every opportunity to write this book. He even taught me how to use the computer. He impressed upon me the fact that there are only twenty-four hours in a day and that this book would make my knowledge available to all the people that I never get a chance to reach.

I would also like to thank Kathy Travers and Mary Beth Hanson for their continued support during the writing of this book. Both kept reminding me of how much an alternative medicine book was needed by pet owners.

Lastly, I could never have sat at the computer all those hours without my three cats and my monkey, Wally. No matter what time it was, all four of them would gather around the desk and stay with their mom until we all went to bed. All of my animals are on my 30-day adult program, and are in purrfect health!

A portion of the proceeds from this book will go to the ASPCA "Coco fund." This is an animal welfare fund designated to help homeless monkeys, large cats (lions, tigers, etc.), and other "exotic" animals that have been taken away from their natural environment and abused by man. Every animal deserves a chance to be happy and healthy.

Introduction

· ·

For as long as I can remember, I have devoted my life to the well-being of animals. I know that the healthier and happier your cat is, the tighter that enormously important human-animal bond can become. I have always felt that it is a veterinarian's job to help owners prevent problems BEFORE they occur (whenever possible), and to help cure them when possible. I have seen frustrated owners deal with unhealthy cats until the very end—giving up after there doesn't seem to be any more hope. It is surmised that many of the hundreds of thousands of cats dumped on the streets or brought to shelters is because of health and/or behavior problems that the owner simply can't live with anymore.

I know that many health and behavioral problems can be overcome without medicine—I've done it for thousands of cats over the years. Your cat's health and attitude is a reflection of its overall nourishment, basic personality, and living conditions. I want to help you keep your cat healthy and happy by teaching you all about nutrition.

It is important that you honestly believe in NUTRITION, which is why I'll start the book with the story of Taschi—my college cat who lived with me all through veterinary school, and then some, and how I found him as a little sickly kitten. Taschi had distemper, a virus that does not respond to antibiotics and is usually fatal. The only hope Taschi had was for me to build up his body's defenses by force-feeding him certain foods, so that he would have a chance to fight off the most dreaded of diseases! That episode of my life convinced me that I had to become a veterinarian, and that nutrition would be my favorite subject. In the first chapter, The Love-Life-Diet Connection, I share some of the case histories of cats who simply could not be cured until I intervened with my favorite medicine—good nutrition. Those cats convinced me, and I hope I will convince you, that nutrition is REALLY IMPORTANT.

While you probably know that dry skin and obesity are nutritional problems and have nutritional solutions, it may surprise you that cancer, allergies, and anxiety can also have nutritional causes and solutions!

The second chapter, Nutritional ABCs for C-A-T-S, teaches you basic nutrition. Cats are not little dogs nor are they little children; they have specific nutritional requirements that I discuss so that you can understand why certain things can be fed to them while others are simply not appropriate! I want you to understand the basic needs of the cat, so that you are not just blindly following directions. I've made the sections on the basic nutrients easy and fun to read. I took each important nutrient, explained what it is, how it benefits your cat, how much you should give your cat (healthy or sick), and the best sources to find that nutrient. To give you an example of how easy this chapter is, let's suppose you want to know about vitamin C. You will see that it's made in the liver of your cat, and that it's needed for tissue repair and helps to stimulate the immune system. It can be used for allergies, viral diseases, such as distemper and leukemia, and is one of the best antioxidants money can buy. The dosage can vary from 100–500 mg depending on what you are using it for. If you don't like to give supplements, you can give your cat vitamin C by giving it bee pollen, green peas, or cantaloupe (you would be surprised at how many cats love fruits and vegetables).

I couldn't write this new book without including the section on Herbs and Other Things. Alfalfa, bee pollen, wheat grass, and acidophillus are just some of the healthy herbs and other things that can help your cat. I have an anxious, loud Siamese-type cat who laps up chamomile tea every afternoon—it's the only way his feline brothers and I can live with him. The chamomile tea takes the edge off his anxiety, and he absolutely loves it, especially if I put it in a glass that allows for easy lapping!

Since antioxidants are the nutrients of the '90s, I had to include a section on them. Once you quickly read that section you will know about other antioxidants besides vitamin C and E and understand why they are so important to your cat's body.

Once I explained the basics on the nutritional components of the diet, I thought it wise to add a chapter titled Must-Knows for Mealtimes. This chapter includes important data that one never seems to have when it's needed; the number of calories a cat needs, how to age your cat, why you should not feed your cat raw meat, and which house plants are not an acceptable food. The last section of the chapter, Life Preventative Nutrition Tactics, will tell you what supplements I recommend for young and old cats.

Let's Talk Cat Food is the food shopping chapter, which discusses the brands of cat food available—what's good and what's bad!

The Feeding for Fitness chapter tells you what a kitten needs to stay healthy, what an adult needs, and, of course, what the senior feline needs. Since I am seeing more and more chubby cats, feeding for weight loss is an important section of this chapter.

Unfortunately, I also see cats with emotional and behavioral problems. Luckily many of these problems have nutritional solutions, which are covered in the corresponding chapters of Getting Emotional and Getting Territorial. Since all cats are different, I found it necessary to have a chapter on Special Needs of Special Breeds and, of course, a chapter devoted to Special Problems.

The chapter titled Getting Physical really puts all of the information together. This is where I have selected the most common problems and their nutritional solutions. It gives you the chance to look up a problem your cat may have and find the nutritional solution. All cats have some type of problem, at one time or another. As an owner you should watch your cat's daily activities so that you can be aware of any problem—hairballs, dry skin, anxiety, just to name a few. Use this section of problems and solutions as a guide to help you adjust your cat's meals and/or supplements. Please note that this section does not replace your family veterinarian—it merely helps to keep you out of his office except for yearly routine examinations and vaccinations.

All this information is designed into a 30-Day Plan for your cat.

It includes diet, exercise and grooming—everything an owner has to do, day by day, for a HEALTHIER AND HAPPIER CAT!

For those of you who don't have time to follow a 30-day plan or read all about nutrition, I have compiled a table of common health and behavioral problems and their nutritional remedies.

There are nutritional dos and don'ts for young, middle-aged, old, and sick cats, which are foundations for your cat's proper health. My book explains these very important fundamentals in an easy-to-understand method. I have even included information for the various purebred cats who may often have some special dietary needs.

Once you understand the basic components of a healthy cat diet, I then evaluate the cat foods sold in the supermarket, pet stores, and veterinary offices, discussing the nutritional components available or absent in the foods. This section allows you to select the cat food that will give your cat what it needs during its particular stage in life (e.g., fat, young and playful, sensitive gastrointestinal tract).

Since store-bought food does not include many other nutritional components, I discuss herbs, vitamins, minerals, and other supplements that can be used for prevention as well as for specific diseases, including cancer, cataracts, arthritis, heart disease, etc.

Finally, after you have the basic understanding of feline nourishment, I put together a 30-day prevention and treatment plan for your cat. This plan is designed to allow you to record your cat's condition one day at a time, throughout the weeks, until the last day. It is tailored to meet the hectic schedule of today's working parents—because it really is simple.

Part One

. . . .

Feeding to Win

. . . .

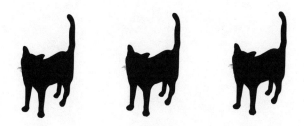

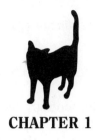

CHAPTER 1

. . . .

The Love-Life-Diet Connection

. . . .

My Love-Life-Diet Discovery

How a sick cat from Brooklyn turned my life around . . .

Though I'd lived with animals all my life, preferred them to playmates of my own species, and from childhood had a special love for cats, I hadn't planned on becoming a veterinarian.

I hadn't planned on a lot of things that were going to change my life.

Luck and Fate: I was a student at the time, living alone in New York, and studying to be a pharmacist. On my way home from class one day, I was walking past an abandoned lot when something stopped me: a faint, pathetically faint, mewling.

I knew at once there was a cat in trouble, but not until I reached her, pushed aside the weeds, and knelt down beside this pitifully emaciated, obviously dehydrated, little orphan Coon cat did I realize how serious the trouble was. She was feverish, her eyes watery and barely open. Her natural black coat with its chest bib of white (barely discernible) was a lifeless, rat-colored gray, matted with excrement and dirt.

The symptoms were frighteningly familiar and heartbreakingly classic: distemper.

I petted her tentatively. Weak as she was, she somehow managed to raise her head and look at me; it was a look of gratitude and a plea for help that I've never forgotten.

Without hesitating, I picked her up and raced to the nearest phone booth. Setting her down gently on my sweater, I grabbed the yellow pages and called the first veterinarian listed. I explained the situation and the kitten's symptoms, and to my dismay was told that nothing could be done and not to bring her in. I got the same response from the next vet I phoned . . . and the next . . . and the next. . . . It wasn't until I reached "veterinary clinics" that a vet finally agreed to see us.

Distemper was accepted routinely in those days—and by many today—as virtually incurable for cats; for kittens it was a death sentence.

The little orphan trying to push her nose against my arm couldn't have been more than two months old.

Wrapping her in my sweater, I ran home for my car, set her tiny, limp body on my lap, and named her Tashi, crooning it as we headed for the clinic.

I felt like crying when we reached the clinic. It was wedged between a butcher shop and a laundromat in a rundown section of Brooklyn. From the outside the place looked more like a flophouse than a veterinary hospital. The waiting room didn't look much better.

Neither did Tashi.

The doctor, Dr. Goldberg, led us into the examining room immediately. Before I'd even put Tashi on the table, he had a syringe in his hand, told me to hold her steady, and gave her an injection. Then he examined her thoroughly, nose to tail, shaking his head sadly throughout the entire procedure.

"Will she . . . ?" I couldn't even ask the question.

"You must force her to eat," he said. It was a command, not advice. "She needs liquids, good nourishment, and food that will harden her stool." He wrote out a short list and handed it to me.

"But—but what about medication? Antibiotics?"

"The last thing this animal needs in her condition is to lose more nutrients. What I've already given her to prevent further dehydration and infection was a risk, not a cure." He sighed. "I'm sorry. What upsets me is, now that vets know that drugs can do many things, they often forget that these are not always the right things to do."

How true, I thought, recalling a test I'd taken recently on the revised indications and contraindications for established medications. But how frustrating. I stared at the list Dr. Goldberg had given me.

He pressed my fingers closed around it. "There is nothing more I can do."

Saying thank you numbly, I cradled Tashi in my arms and asked what I owed.

"You are a student, yes?"

I nodded.

"You owe me nothing."

"Nothing?" Stunned and grateful, I thanked him again. I had no idea at that time how very much I owed him.

As I turned to leave, he said, "Bring her back tomorrow if she's still alive."

Night Shift: I spent nearly that entire evening hand-feeding Tashi at regular intervals, giving her teaspoons of professional cat food (discussed in chapter 4) blended with pureed, cooked chicken livers and rice and what I calculated from my basic pharmaceutical and nutritional training would be a balanced amount of pediatric vitamins and minerals for her age and size. Using an eyedropper, I was also able to give her a mixture of diluted evaporated milk, honey, and raw egg yolk.

Now, for a healthy kitten this would have been royal treatment beyond belief: constant attention, specially prepared finger-fed gourmet food, and all accompanied by delicious milk and honey.

Unfortunately, Tashi was anything but a healthy kitten. Having distemper disease—known for causing cats to refuse to eat or drink and therefore, unwittingly starving them to death—she seemed to view my nutritional ministrations as cruel and unusual punishment. This broke my heart, yet I couldn't really blame her.

What I've euphemistically described as hand-feeding was actually force-feeding (which does have a sort of cruel-and-unusual-punishment ring to it). Nonetheless, it is a technique that's often required for a cat's well-being. In Tashi's case it was a matter of life or death. And I was determined not to settle for the latter.

I ignored her feeble protests and sustained myself by repeating, "All's fair in love and war" and that this was war and I was in love.

Somewhere around 5 A.M. battle fatigue set in.

Tashi, for all my ministrations, had evidenced no improvement. Exhausted, disheartened, and inconsolably sad, I fell asleep beside her. I didn't want to think about waking up.

Three hours later, I had no choice: two white-tipped paws were patting my nose, a black tail was tickling my chin, and a warm furry head was rubbing against my chest. I was euphoric. She'd made it through the night.

I couldn't wait to call Dr. Goldberg.

That afternoon, when he'd completed examining Tashi, Dr. Goldberg once again shook his head sadly and said exactly what he'd said the day before, and would continue to say for the next week: "Bring her in tomorrow if she's still alive."

I did—and she became more alive with each passing day.

An Ending and a Beginning: Within four weeks the scrawny Brooklyn back-lot orphan—now savoring my specially prepared meals and thriving—blossomed into a five-pound bundle of boundless energy and remarkable beauty, and, along with Dr. Goldberg, changed the course of my life forever: I no longer wanted to be a pharmacist—I was determined to be a veterinarian.

Tashi and I enjoyed many wonderful years together, both here and in Italy, where I graduated summa cum laude from veterinary school. Her special combination of feline mischief and magic was unique, and though I've loved and lived with many cats, I never will or can forget her.

Nor will or can I ever forget Dr. Goldberg, that wonderful man who always insisted I owed him nothing, but whose unconventional forays into the curative and preventive powers of nutrients have been—and still are—a continuing inspiration for dedicating my veterinary career to animal nutrition.

Tails That Told More Than Stories

There's no pussyfooting around nutrition when you're catering to cats.

As a veterinarian at the County Animal Clinic in Yonkers, New York, I was one of a fortunate few privileged to have daily contact and consultation with some of the nation's foremost board-certified specialists in all fields of animal medicine. It was an incomparable opportunity for gaining firsthand, state-of-the-art veterinary experience, opening vast areas of knowledge to me, particularly about felines, and was essentially responsible for my realization that most sick cats are victims of uneducated owners or casualties of ill-equipped boarding facilities.

Convinced of this, Dr. Richard Jackimer (also from the County Animal Clinic) and veterinary technician Chris Thedings joined me in opening the Cat Hilt-Inn. It was the first four-star feline boarding facility owned and operated by registered veterinarians, totally dedicated to maximizing the health of all cat residents through nutrition.

My enthusiasm for the endeavor was boundless. And though it cost me nights of sleep, days of frustration, and incalculable hours of work, what I learned from our boarders and their owners was priceless.

The Mysteriously Balding Siamese Siblings

Maja and Raja were two six-year-old Siamese cats who had never been boarded before. Their owners had been called to England to settle some family affairs and would be unable to return for at least a month. They were distraught about leaving their "babies."

I was distraught looking at their "babies."

Though the animals' health forms (required for all cats we boarded) appeared to be in order, Maja and Raja certainly did not. Both were virtually hairless and had chests so slack and saggy they resembled kangaroo pouches. Talk about an undynamic duo! This pair exhibited about as much vitality as a couple of garden slugs. Something was definitely wrong.

I had nothing to go on but a hunch, so I decided to play it: I asked what the cats were being fed.

"Only the best!" I was told indignantly.

"Only the best what?" I asked, soft-pedaling my tone of voice so as not to appear dubious.

"Ground steak and raw liver."

"And . . . ?" I prompted, waiting for them to continue.

"And nothing else," was their defiant reply.

My hunch had been right. Maja and Raja were suffering from a royal case of all-meat syndrome, a completely unbalanced diet that was not only denying but depleting them of essential nutrients (particularly B vitamins and carbohydrates), causing them increasing loss of energy and general deteriorating health.

I requested permission to change Maja and Raja's diet to a balanced-formula cat food. Well . . . you would have thought I'd asked to feed them cyanide! I was told in no uncertain terms that their "babies" would never eat it.

It took me awhile to get the owners' approval, but after I assured them that the new diet would be given on a carefully supervised trial basis and that the cats would never go hungry, they reluctantly consented. (They were convinced, I'm sure, that they were never going to see Maja and Raja again.) I promised to send a letter every week, keeping them informed of their pets' condition.

They left teary-eyed and forlorn.

That night I gave Maja and Raja each a bowl of dry, professional, fixed-formula food, high in recuperative and bodybuilding nutrients. Let me just say, for animals who "would never eat cat food," those two did a superb job of faking it. They devoured every morsel and continued to do so for all the days that followed.

Within one week their hair began to grow back; within two, their coats were fine-textured and glossy, and with daily exercise their kangaroo pouches were beginning to firm into muscles. By the third week they were looking sleek and growing more energetic daily. By the end of their four-week stay, they were the Hilt-Inn's most glamorous, mischievous, and talkative couple (if it was time for dinner, they let me know it!).

When their owners returned, they viewed Maja and Raja's transformation as nothing less than a miracle, even though I explained that it was nothing more than nutrition. They didn't care. Maja and Raja were signed on as regular weekend boarders.

MORAL: *Food that is "only the best" for people can be just about the worst for cats.*

The Cat with Invisible Legs

She was an orange tabby named Goldilocks and looked as if she'd just eaten three bears. Obese? This cat made Garfield look anorectic.

She was so fat that when she stood (which was in itself a remarkable feat), her legs were invisible, totally hidden by her enormous body.

Since Goldilocks also had a rash that extended from midback to tail, had cowlicks of matted fur, and reeked of unpleasant fecal odor, I immediately asked what she was being fed.

"Well, I like to treat her kind of special," replied the owner. "She has a tendency to be frightened and pants a lot, so I guess I sort of spoil her." She then proceeded to tell me that she not only left three varieties of dry food available for Goldilocks at all times, but gave her breakfast leftovers, luncheon leftovers, a can of 9 Lives for dinner, and a bedtime snack of whatever pastry, pudding, or ice cream happened to be around (judging from the owner's own more than ample figure, I suspected these were rarely not around). This woman was not spoiling her cat, she was killing it. Goldilocks's frightened panting was due, I felt certain, to excess fat around her heart.

"She's quite a bit overweight," I said as tactfully as possible.

"Goldie?" The woman shook her head. "She's just a big cat; eats everything I give her." No doubt about that, I thought, but felt it inappropriate to say so at the time.

As the woman rose to leave, it took several moments for her to lift Goldilocks and plump all twenty-seven pounds of her into my lap. "You know," she said, slightly winded, "maybe Goldie could lose a little weight."

That's what I wanted to hear.

The first night with Goldilocks was the hardest. I started her on Feline r/d, a professional reducing diet cat food that supplied all necessary nutrients and included enough bulk fiber to appease her hunger without adding calories.

I weighed her every day, and by the end of the first week she had lost two pounds and was beginning to groom herself (which was almost physically impossible at her former size, especially with that enormous belly). After losing two more pounds the following week, Goldilocks really got into the grooming. The rash on her back began to clear up, because she was using her tongue regularly to clear away dead epithelial cells, stimulate her oil glands, and distribute her natural oils. Her cowlicks disappeared and her fur began to shine.

Within three weeks she was visibly slimmer, more alert, more active, and odor-free, since she now could easily clean her anal-genital area.

The owner was ecstatic when she saw the change in Goldilocks's appearance, and promised she would keep up the food and grooming regiment I'd begun. I told her to brush Goldilocks daily with a soft (natural bristle) brush, weigh her daily, and keep her on the reducing diet for at least another month or two, then switch to a good alternative food.

She obviously followed my instructions, because when I saw them some time later, Goldilocks was in grand condition. She was still chubby—and most likely always would be—but she was outgoing, healthy, and strutting on four now very visible legs. Probably not coincidentally, the owner had dropped some weight and looked much better, too.

MORAL: *Cats given too many treats get unjust desserts.*

The Scaredy-Cat Solution

Oscar was a slim, lethargic, dull-gray, pin-striped, domestic shorthair around six years old. His owner had brought him in for boarding because she was upset about his increasing timidity, aversion to socializing, and general apathy. She believed Oscar had a psychological problem.

When I asked why she believed this (since the cat had been heard and seen playing while she was at work), she explained that several years before, Oscar, who's always been essentially an indoor cat (with limited yard privileges in summer), had witnessed a neighbor's cat kill a bird and eat it. She was convinced that this had traumatized Oscar and was the cause of her formerly outgoing, active pet's current introverted behavior.

I found it difficult to share her conviction. For one cat to see another kill a bird could hardly be construed as traumatic, particularly since hunting and prey-catching are innate in felines, even if they've never been outside. Whatever Oscar's problem, that wasn't it.

I looked over his admittance form and saw nothing unusual. But I had learned from past experience that much of what wasn't written turned out to be what was most informative. And more often than not—as I was discovering daily—that information had to do with diet. I asked about Oscar's.

"Well, he always has dry food available," his owner told me, "but he gets a can of food for breakfast before I go to work, then another can for dinner when I come home, and then before I go to bed I give him, you know, some sort of treat. A muffin, a piece of pie, cookies, whatever's around. And he eats all of it."

I was surprised and slightly baffled. That amount of food was excessive, even for the most active cat, and yet Oscar was not overweight. A former extrovert, he had now regressed to curling up behind chairs and under the bed. The pieces didn't seem to fit, but I had more than a sneaking suspicion that they would. I asked her to leave Oscar with me for the week.

I put Oscar on a normal twice-a-day feeding schedule, and within three days discovered through a routine fecal examination that his ravenous appetite and lack of weight gain were due to tapeworms. His assumed timidity, aversion to socializing, and lethargy had come about simply because his owner was serving him a feline equivalent of three Thanksgiving dinners daily! No wonder he didn't care to do more than just lie down and curl up. Who would? Who could?

I explained this to his owner, though she was still reluctant to concede that Oscar's problem was not psychological until she came to pick him up, and he obliterated all doubt by literally bounding into her arms. After a week of having been fed just two quality meals a day—and in spite of not yet being completely worm-free—his timidity and apathy were gone. High-spirited, extroverted Oscar was back to normal and raring to go.

MORAL: *Never overfeed a cat with anything but love.*

Making Your Own Discoveries

Your lack of curiosity could be harmful to your cat.

Once a cat has become established as an integral part of your home and your life, it's not uncommon for both of you to take each other for granted, especially where feeding is concerned. This is perfectly understandable. After all, it's a routine with seductive, mutual benefits.

For kitty: same food, same time, same place; dependable.

For you: can opener, cup; no thought required.

Unfortunately, these mutual benefits, as with most seductive things, can be risky and have regrettable, unforeseen consequences.

Just because your cat isn't visibly ill doesn't mean that he or she is healthy. I say this not to frighten you, but to impress upon you the amazing fact that the majority of all common cat ailments are preventable and curable through early symptom recognition and the immediate implementation of enhanced immunity nutrition.

Q&A

Jekyll and Hyde Eating

My three-year-old male cat, Rocky (a neutered domestic shorthair), is sort of a Jekyll and Hyde eater. He'll devour half a can of Kal Kan's Mealtime in the morning, then won't even touch the other half when I serve it at night, though if I open a can of another food, he'll down it with gusto. Sometimes he'll eat a meal only at night, sometimes just in the morning— and sometimes not at all. I know the food isn't spoiled because I refrigerate it. Have you ever heard of this sort of food neurosis? And is it curable?

I've heard of it: cold-food neurosis. Happily, it's not really a neurosis and is readily curable. Rocky, not unlike many cats, just doesn't like cold food. (This isn't an unwise preference on his part, since cold food often causes gastric disturbances in cats.) I'd suggest warming the refrigerated portions of his meals to room temperature. Either add a tablespoon of hot water or broth, mix, then test with your finger; warm the can in hot water as you would a baby bottle; or remove the contents to a microwave dish and warm. Be careful to mix the food well and test to make sure your cat doesn't burn his tongue. Never reheat the food. This destroys the nutrients and will make the meal worthless for feeding.

One alternative (though it could be costly) is to buy smaller, one-portion cans; another is to feed Rocky a quality low-magnesium-content dry food. (See chapters 4 and 11 for suggestions.)

Flaky Cat

I have a black shorthaired house cat with a dandruff problem. She's been checked for worms and has none. I bathe and brush her regularly, but it doesn't seem to help. I tried adding bacon grease to her food, but it made her vomit, so I stopped. Any suggestions?

Quite a few. First, hold off on the bathing (shampoos can wash away your cat's natural oils, and unless there is a real need to bathe a cat, don't), but do keep up the brushing. This stimulates oil glands and distributes natural oils. Use a soft bristle brush. Since your cat stays indoors, her skin is more prone to dryness. In winter a humidifier can help, but adjusting her diet is your best all-year-round preventive.

Make sure she is getting an adequate amount of high-quality protein and essential fatty acids—those that cannot be made in the body and must be obtained from food. (See chapter 2.) She also needs ample amounts of vitamin E to prevent oxidation of these fats and to ensure the effectiveness of other fat-soluble vitamins such as A, D, and K as well as B complex.

Avoid feeding all-fish foods, which are high in unsaturated fats that can decrease vitamin E efficiency, and chlorinated water, if possible. Raw egg yolk—not whites—is a good dietary addition, as is any quality fatty-acid supplement (such as Opticoat II, Dr. Jane® Essential Gel, or Linatone).

CHAPTER 2

....

Nutritional ABCs for C-A-T-S

....

While it's not essential that you read this chapter in its entirety (you may just look up the nutritional components that you want to know about), I recommend that you do so. It will give you a solid foundation, which will allow you to better understand the reasons behind some of my recommendations. This chapter includes facts about proteins, fats and carbohydrates. These food groups are explained in a light and easy manner, but with enough information to give you a real feel for basic nutrition. I explain the differences between proteins and why some fats are better than others. Fiber, a carbohydrate, is one of the hottest items in nutritional science. Fiber plays an important role in maintaining a healthy gut, and will be used throughout the book in sections concerning diarrhea, constipation, and diabetes. The brief summary given in this chapter will help you understand why certain fibers are being recommended for specific problems, as opposed to other fibers.

Vitamins and minerals are certainly another hot topic of discussion, especially antioxidants. To supplement or not to supplement, and if so, which vitamins and/or minerals should be given? Every vitamin and mineral is explained briefly, including how it benefits your cat, how much should be given to a healthy cat or sick cat, and which food(s) naturally contain a specific vitamin or mineral in case you would rather use a natural source instead of a prepared supplement.

"Whole foods" (which include herbs, bee pollen, seaweeds and various grasses) are the sources of many of these vitamins, minerals, proteins, fats, and carbohydrates, and are one of the safest ways to supplement. As you will see in this chapter, you can overdose with vitamins and minerals, but rarely with herbs! If you are feeding with a professional alternative food, it can be unwise to add a vitamin, multivitamins and/or minerals; these can easily throw off the balance of that expensive, well-formulated food. Yet, I believe that our commercial cat foods need to be supplemented. Feline nutrition is a young science, and we are just learning about the needs of cats. Over the last ten years, the pet food industry has revised the requirements for many well-known food components, adding more or deleting where necessary, but commercial foods still have a long way to go.

Taurine is one of those food components that most cat foods simply didn't have in sufficient amounts. Manufacturers, veterinarians, and owners had no idea that the "Complete and Balanced" food was lacking this essential amino acid until, by luck, a scientist happened to piece together the incidences of heart disease, blindness, and the lack of taurine in the cat's blood. It seems that when the manufacturers did not use ingredients naturally abundant in taurine and supplemented what they believed was enough taurine to the food, some of the additional taurine was being destroyed in the cooking, leaving many cats taurine-deficient. This deficiency showed up as heart disease and/or blindness. The cat food manufacturers have since elevated their minimum requirements for this amino acid that natural cat food (mice) contains in sufficient amounts. The taurine lesson demonstrates that we can't be sure that the food is 100 percent balanced, especially for your cat, since every cat has different needs.

Herbal medicine is returning after thousands of years. Garlic was used as an antibiotic, long before penicillin was used or known about, and for repelling fleas for centuries. Today, garlic is again being used as an aid in combatting fleas, and it's recommended for certain diseases. I've included the herbs that I find the easiest to give to a cat and those which are the most effective. They can be used medicinally or as preventive supplements. My cats get Dr. Jane® Beezme, a combination of bee pollen and vegetable enzymes, as *the* daily supplement of choice, replacing synthetic multivitamin/mineral supplements.

Bee pollen, one of the oldest complete foods in the world, is giving my cats nutritional components that simply are not found in corn, rice, chicken, fish or any of the common ingredients that cat food manufacturers use today. Scientists are looking closely at bee pollen and other herbs and studying all their different components to learn their natural secrets so that those new components can be synthetically prepared and sold to the public. As they isolate nutrient by nutrient, they are finding that the nutrients work best when they are in combination, just as in nature—not when they are individually given to the animal. I predict that herbs will become the favorite new supplements, and that my herbal section will give you a jump start on it all!

Why Human and Cat Nutritional Needs Differ

*Our brains are similar, but our
dietary needs are not.*

Except for our larger frontal lobes and speech and memory-association capacities, cats and humans have virtually identically structured brains. This is a fine bit of trivia, but useless—and often harmful—when it comes to eating, feeding and nutrition.

Your Cat Is Not a Little Furry Person: No matter how human your cat behaves, whether it licks your ear like a lover, demands hors d'oeuvres at cocktail parties, is easily insulted, has opinions about your friends, or cons you into giving up your place on the couch, its digestive system, metabolism, and nutrient needs are uniquely feline.

Differences That Make the Difference

- Protein requirements for cats are higher than those for humans.
- Cats, unlike humans (or dogs and other mammals), cannot

store excess protein and must replenish their supply through daily dietary intake.

- Cats cannot be vegetarians and thrive; they have short intestines, whereas humans have long ones, and therefore cats are unable to utilize vegetable protein effectively. Moreover, cats cannot convert beta-carotene, present in plants, to vitamin A (even though beta-carotene still has antioxidant effects). Cats must get their vitamin A from meat-animal tissue.
- Taurine is essential to cats—they can't make it. Cats, unlike humans and dogs, must have meat proteins (fish included) to get their daily requirement of taurine, an amino acid that they cannot make, but must ingest. Deficiency causes blindness, heart disease and reproduction problems.
- Growing kittens need about one-third more protein per pound than do human infants.
- An eleven-pound cat needs approximately the same daily minimum of thirty grams of protein that a forty-four-pound, four- to six-year-old child does!
- Cats must consume the preformed arachidonic fatty acid found only in animal tissues, since, unlike humans, they cannot convert linoleic or arachidonic fatty acid. (See "Fats.")
- Cats can have diets consisting of up to 64 percent fat (and I mean the kind of saturated fat that doctors tell us to cut down on or die) and live healthier and more vigorous lives than the majority of nutrition-conscious humans.
- Magnesium dosages that help humans prevent kidney stones can create them in cats, along with FLUTD (feline lower urological disease syndrome) and other bladder and kidney ailments.
- Humans can use the amino acid tryptophan to manufacture the B vitamin niacin, but cats cannot, and therefore cats need more niacin in their diet.

PROTEIN
The Number-One Cat Nutrient

What It Is

- Protein is the foremost dietary structural material for all mammals in general, and cats in particular.
- Protein is a combination of amino acids—the building blocks of protein—that form thousands of different proteins (which perform specific functions) and are also the end product of protein digestion.
- The essential amino acids cats must obtain from foods are:

arginine	*phenylalanine*	*histidine*	*taurine*
isoleucine	*threonine*	*leucine*	*tryptophan*
lysine	*valine*	*methionine*	

Benefits

- Helps growth, maintenance, and repair of all animal tissue.
- Promotes and sustains a high-powered immunity system.
- Fuels the active feline metabolism.
- Aids in developing and strengthening a cat's thousands of springlike muscles. (Building muscles requires exercise by cats as well as humans.)

How Much Is Needed?

Adult cats need 3 g per pound of body weight daily. Kittens need 8.6 g per pound of body weight daily.
Remember: Cats cannot store excess protein and must replenish their supply every day through food.

Sources

Lean muscle meat (beef, lamb, turkey, chicken); fish (cooked); egg yolk (no uncooked whites); whole egg (cooked); organ meats (kidney, liver); whole milk (protein casein); torula or brewer's yeast, bee pollen, and wheat germ.

Deficiency Symptoms and Diseases

Abdomen distension (swollen belly); hair loss; lethargy; dry, brittle hair, whiskers, and nails.

Advice

Whoever said "You can't get too much of a good thing," does not know enough about cat nutrition. As important a nutrient as protein is, it should not be your cat's entire diet. All-meat or all-fish diets cause more harm than health! In fact, even though pregnant and lactating cats, as well as growing kittens, need increased protein in their diets, feeding them only meat can cause calcium deficiencies.

Remember that the protein you do feed your cat should be as complete as possible; that is, it should contain as many of the essential amino acids, if not all of them. Since cereals lack essential amino acids, feed animal protein.

Always bear in mind that the better the protein quality—"quality" meaning its high biological value (BV) and efficient usability by the body—the less your cat needs. Protein percentages on labels are often misleading and can undermine your pet's health if read incorrectly. An egg has a biological value of 100%. That means that it contains every needed amino acid, even though they are not in the required amounts. Corn meal has a biological value of approximately 60%. Meat generally has a higher biological value than plant protein. Meat by-products (kidney, liver, heart) have a high value, while other by-products (feet, intestines) can have very low values. The protein percentages on a can or bag of food can, therefore, be meaningless. A percentage does not reflect the TYPE of protein, and therefore its usage by the body. A leather shoe can be 100% protein, but is certainly not usable!

Therefore, don't read ONLY the percentages; look for the meat ingredients.

CARBOHYDRATES

What They Are

- Carbohydrates are nutrients derived from plants.
- Carbohydrates include starches, sugars, cereals, and plant fiber.

Benefits

As long as your cat is getting a proper protein/fat ratio in its diet, the right carbohydrates can serve as a backup energy source.

Fiber, such as bran or beet pulp:
- provides necessary bulk to stimulate intestinal movement, prevents constipation and firms stools.
- helps cleanse intestine walls of digested food residue (chyme).
- forms a gel in the gastrointestinal tract that regulates the absorption of nutrients, particularly water and minerals, taurine and sugar.
- provides the intestinal cells with essential nutrients for their health.

How Much Is Needed?

Cats have no standard requirements for carbohydrates, but for optimal health they need at least one—processed rice, corn, or wheat (not whole)—and preferably two, for backup energy.

Not more than 10 to 15 percent of a cat's daily diet should consist of carbohydrates.

Amount of fiber is best determined by an individual cat's needs (too little: constipation; too much: diarrhea).

Sources

For backup energy: processed corn, wheat, barley or rice. For fiber: wheat bran, beet pulp, vegetables, and fruit. For diarrhea management: brown watery cooked rice, beet pulp, plants containing a special type of carbohydrate (F.O.S.) that balances the intestinal bacteria population (avocado).

Deficiency Symptoms and Diseases

None known, though chronic constipation could indicate a deficiency of fiber.

Propolyn glycol, a sugar, can destroy red blood cells.

Advice

Many cats enjoy raw vegetables and fruits (my cat, Orisha, adores alfalfa sprouts, peas, and avocados) and benefit from the vitamins, minerals, and fiber they contain. These vegetarian indulgences are fine as long as your cat's primary diet has an ample protein/fat content.

Vegetarians and dieters take heart: if your cat is into veggies, there's nothing wrong with having your pet join you in a salad once or twice a month. Indoor cats love it!

Raw starches can often cause diarrhea in cats, which is why grains and legumes should be cooked and ground, so that the carbohydrates they contain can be digested.

If you want the benefits of fiber for your cat, wheat or rice bran will provide the kind you're looking for. An oatmeal breakfast recipe can be a great early morning treat. A pot of wheat grass is a healthy, high-fiber snack.

FATS

What They Are

- Fats are the most concentrated source of a cat's dietary energy. (Fat contains approximately twice the calories of either carbohydrates or protein.) When fats are hard, they are called fats, and when they are liquid, they are called oils.
- Fats are composed of fatty acids; those of prime importance for your cat are linoleic, linolenic, and arachidonic. These unsaturated fatty acids are called "essential," because they cannot be manufactured by the cat's body and must be obtained through diet. Linoleic and linolenic can come from vegetable sources,

but arachidonic acid must be obtained from animal fat and must be obtained through diet.

- They form the vitamins F, A, D, E and K (fat-soluble vitamins) around the body and enable them to be properly utilized.
- Their quality and type are more important than their percentage in your cat's diet.

Benefits

- Makes foods more palatable.
- Supplies needed energy, particularly during periods of growth or stress.
- Promotes healthy skin and shiny coat.
- Aids in feline fitness by regulating glandular activity and making calcium readily available to cells.
- Helps improve immunity in tissue.
- Assists in thermal regulation of body temperature.

How Much Is Needed?

A balanced dry food should not contain less than 15 percent fat.

The average house cat's daily diet should contain 20 to 40 percent fat.

As much as 64 percent of your cat's caloric needs can be given in the form of fat, unless obesity is a problem. (See chapter 11.)

The AAFCO feline nutritional requirements list 0.5% linoleic acid and .02% arachidonic acid for growth, reproduction, and adult maintenance as the minimum amount of fat needed. This does not take into consideration different types of fats, nor the individual requirements of cats.

Sources

Soft animal fat (chicken fat, bacon grease); butter; fish oils; flax seed oil.

Linoleic, linolenic fatty acids: vegetable oils (i.e., corn); fish oil; borage oil; flax seed oil.

Symptoms and Diseases

Dry skin (itching and scratching); lethargy; reproduction problems; and frequent illness.

Advice

In order to evaluate pet food, you need to know the difference between soft fats and hard fats. Soft fats are, essentially, those that melt easily (for example, poultry fat, butter, bacon grease, and lard). These are extremely beneficial to your cat because they are readily digested and are able to supply energy as well as to quickly carry vitamins A and E, choline, and other nutrients where they're needed.

Because of their availability and low cost, hard fats are often used in cat food. If properly processed and cleanly rendered, they are fine sources of arachidonic acid, which cats cannot synthesize and must obtain from animal fats. A label may or may not denote the type of fat used. While some manufacturers use the word "chicken fat," others will use "animal fat," which can be either hard or soft, chicken, or tallow. I would call the manufacturer and ask what type is used. Generally speaking if the manufacturer doesn't name the fat specifically, then it usually indicates tallow, a hard fat.

Unusable fat usually goes one of five places: (1) It's vomited; (2) it's stored in the liver, killing cells, and could eventually cause fatty liver disease; (3) it becomes adipose tissue (tummy fat); (4) it goes out the oil glands (you have one greasy cat); or (5) it passes through the stool. So when you think of adding fat to your cat's diet, do your pet a favor and think "soft" in small quantities.

Although the addition of a little chicken fat never hurt any cat, if you feel that your cat needs additional fat (for coat and skin, for calories, or to enhance the immune system), your best bet is to buy a balanced "fatty acid" supplement. These contain the correct ratios of fatty acids with their necessary vitamins and minerals.

Be aware of "all natural." The manufacturer might not have added anything, but the fat supplier or the vitamin supplier may have already added chemical preservatives. If the cat food manufacturer did not add preservatives themselves, then they do not have to put them on the label even though they may be in the food tied to the fat or fat-soluble vitamins. Thus, many manufacturers are preserving fats with vitamin E (mixed tocopherols), and/or C and rosemary, and the food may still contain preservatives. If a product contains any artificial preservatives from the vitamins, then the package must not only say "natural" but it must also say "fortified with vitamins and minerals."

Keep in mind that chemically preserved food is not necessarily bad! Rancidity causes all types of problems from poor skin and coat and abnormal bone growth to a possibility of cancer! Some people claim their cats are "allergic" to artificial preservatives. Their stories blame all types of diseases, even cancer, on them. The truth is, a cat may be sensitive to a preservative, but no one has proven that preservatives actually cause allergy—and there has been no evidence to support any negative claims.

VITAMINS

Vitamins are organic substances found in minute quantities in natural food and are essential to normal life-functioning in all animals. With few exceptions they cannot be manufactured internally and must be obtained through diet or supplements.

VITAMIN A

What It Is

- It is a fat-soluble vitamin that requires sufficient fats and minerals in order for proper absorption to take place.
- Though there are two forms of this vitamin—preformed vitamin A (called retinol and found only in foods of animal origin) and provitamin A (called beta-carotene and found primarily in foods of plant origin)—cats, unlike humans and dogs, can not convert beta-carotene to vitamin A and must obtain it from retinol (an animal source). Beta-carotene is an antioxidant and does not have to be converted to vitamin A for its antioxidant effect.

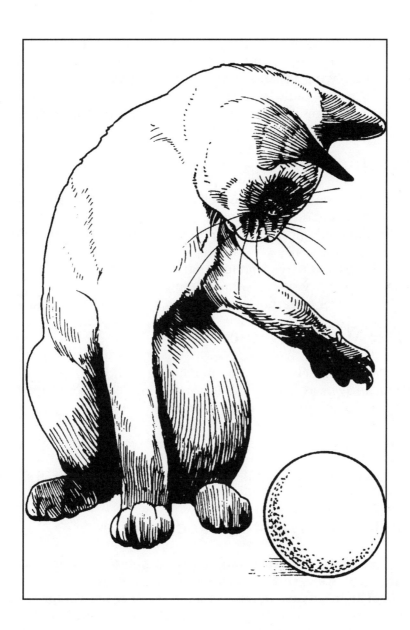

- As a fat-soluble vitamin, it can be stored in the cat's body. Because of this, cats don't need daily replenishment, and an oversupply (for instance, lavishing too much beef liver upon your pet) can cause an unhealthy buildup and hypervitaminosis (symptoms: reduced, painful, or crippling neck movement; abnormal walking; muscle degeneration).

Benefits

- Increases immunity and aids in prevention of bladder, respiratory, and other infections.
- Promotes growth, skin and coat health, fertility, and muscle coordination.
- Helps pituitary gland function.
- Improves vision, hearing, and digestion.
- Provides protection against toxic chemicals in foods and water.

How Much Is Needed?

The recommended minimum daily allowance is 1,000 to 3,000 IU for an average, healthy cat. Because of its potential toxicity, I prefer that you supplement with beta-carotene.

Sources

Liver, kidneys, egg yolk (no uncooked whites), butter, fish liver oil.

Deficiency Symptoms and Diseases

Loss of appetite (anorexia), muscle atrophy, weight loss, dull or brittle coat, scaly hairless patches on skin, overgrowth of the cornea, conjunctivitis, retinal degeneration, intolerance of light (photophobia), resistance to petting or handling, and impaired fertility. In tomcats: testicular atrophy. In kittens: weakness, irregular muscle coordination (ataxia), tremors, and paralysis.

Advice

Vitamin A is vital in the diet of every cat, so be sure it's listed on the label for whatever food you're feeding. And while you're reading that label, check to see that the food doesn't contain sodium nitrate. This additive, present in many cat foods, can deplete vitamin A.

If you're thinking of supplementing your pet's diet, liver is a good choice, but don't overdo it! Too much vitamin A is as dangerous for your cat as too little. I'd suggest that if you're going to add it to your cat's regular food, liver should not make up more than 25 percent of the meal. If you're going to serve liver as a meal in itself, I'd recommend not doing so more than three times a week, unless your veterinarian has specifically advised you to do so.

While cod liver oil is a great source of vitamin A, I don't want you to add it to your cat's diet. Most cat foods, supermarket and alternative, have MORE than enough vitamin A, and that little amount you add may be toxic! If you feel that you want to add additional fat to your cat's diet (besides table scraps), ask your veterinarian for a fat supplement that is appropriate for your cat. A well-made supplement should include linoleic acid, linolenic acid, vitamin E, zinc, biotin and selenium. If the supplement also contains arachidonic acid, that is even better!

If you are looking for an antioxidant, use beta-carotene.

B_1
Thiamine

What It Is

- B_1 is a water-soluble member of the B complex; any excess is excreted instead of being stored in the cat's body and must be replaced daily.
- Cooking heat, food-processing methods, extended storage, sulfa drugs, air and water destroy its potency.
- It works synergistically: it is more effective when taken together with other B vitamins, particularly B_2 (riboflavin) and B_6 (pyridoxine), than alone.

- Cats have an exceptionally high requirement for B complex vitamins.

Benefits

- Stimulates appetite.
- Keeps nervous system, muscles, and heart functioning normally.
- Helps maintain optimal feline fitness.
- Improves mental attitude, behavior, and intelligence.

How Much Is Needed?

The recommended minimum daily allowance is 0.2–1.5 mg for an average, healthy cat. (More is required during lactation, illness, and growth and stress periods.)

Sources

Brewer's yeast, torula yeast, fish, organ meat, asparagus, wheat germ, and bee pollen.

Deficiency Symptoms and Diseases

Loss of appetite (anorexia), loss of muscular coordination (ataxia), vomiting, weight loss, heart dysfunction, convulsions, and paralysis.

Advice

Let me start by telling you to stop feeding your cat raw fish. Many fish, such as carp and herring, contain an element in their tissues that prevents the absorption of thiamine, which can result in your pet developing a vitamin B_1 deficiency.

Because cats have a great need for thiamine (as well as the other B complex vitamins), mix brewer's yeast or torula yeast into their food on a regular basis. Use torula yeast if FLUTD (feline lower urological disease syndrome) is a problem. Not only can this help ensure that cats get their daily requirement, but it can also help keep them flea-free! Thiamine (ample in yeast) seems to give cats some imperceptible scent that repels fleas. (It takes at least a month for this internal repellent to become effective, so don't be disheartened if at first the fleas succeed; brewer's or torula yeast will eventually win—for most cats—especially if you add garlic.

If your cat is on antibiotics, recovering from surgery or under any sort of stress, the need for thiamine (and all B vitamins) is increased. You can use B complex supplements, brewer's or torula yeast, or Pet Ag's Bene Bac (which contains all the B vitamins as well as vitamins A, D, E and acidophilus), available at pet food stores or from your veterinarian.

B_2
Riboflavin

What It Is

- This is another water-soluble member of the B complex, which cannot be stored in your cat's body and needs to be replaced regularly through diet.
- It is easily absorbed and easily excreted.
- Depending on your cat's needs or deficiencies, excretion may be accompanied by protein loss.
- It is not destroyed by heat or oxidation (as thiamine is), but does dissolve in cooking liquids and is destroyed by light.

Benefits

- Helps prevent eye problems and cataracts.
- Aids in metabolization of carbohydrates, protein and fat (essential for the release of energy from food).
- Prevents dry, cracking skin.
- Needed during pregnancy.

How Much Is Needed?

The recommended minimum daily allowance is 0.2–1.5 mg for an average, healthy cat. (More is needed during lactation, illness, and stress or growth periods, and for cats on a high-fat diet.)

Sources

Chicken liver, kidney, cottage cheese, cooked fish, brewer's yeast, milk, asparagus, avocado, torula yeast, and bee pollen.

Deficiency Symptoms and Diseases

Loss of appetite (anorexia), weight loss, cataracts, and hair loss (alopecia). In tomcats: testicular atrophy.

Advice

If your pet is under stress (a move, an operation, an illness), riboflavin, along with the other B complex vitamins and vitamin C, is a wise diet supplement. When adding any of the food sources that I've mentioned above, don't go overboard. These foods should constitute no more than 25 percent of your cat's regular meal, unless your veterinarian has advised you otherwise.

CAUTION: If your cat has cancer and is taking an antineoplastic (anti-cancer) medication, an excess of vitamin B_2 can reduce the drug's effectiveness. Check with your veterinarian before making any diet alterations.

B_3
Niacin, Niacinamide, Nicotinic Acid

What It Is

- Another water-soluble member of the B complex, B_3 needs to be replaced in your cat's daily diet.

- This is easily destroyed by cooking, food processing, sulfa drugs, and water.
- Unlike humans and dogs, cats cannot convert the amino acid tryptophan (found in turkey, meat, cottage cheese) to form niacin, making them completely dependent on dietary intake.
- This is necessary for proper synthesis of insulin, sex hormones, cortisone, and thyroxine (the hormone produced by the thyroid gland).

Benefits

- Increases energy through effectively metabolizing protein and fat.
- Helps prevent negative behavior by promoting a healthy nervous system.
- Aids in eliminating and preventing mouth sores and bad breath.
- Alleviates gastrointestinal problems and keeps digestive system healthy.

How Much Is Needed?

The recommended minimum daily allowance is 2.6–7 mg for an average, healthy cat. (More is needed during lactation, illness, and stress periods.)

CAUTION: Do not give your cat a niacin supplement without a veterinarian's advice. It can cause itching and great discomfort to your pet.

Sources

Liver, heart, kidney, brewer's yeast, torula yeast, poultry white meat, wheat germ, and egg yolk (no uncooked whites).

Deficiency Symptoms and Diseases

Diarrhea, mouth ulcers, thick saliva, bad breath, and fever. In kittens and young cats: loss of appetite (anorexia), weight loss, lethargy, dangerously increased susceptibility to respiratory infections.

Advice

If your cat is taking antibiotics, you might want to add some niacin-rich food to the animal's regular diet. Brewer's yeast (unless FLUTD is a problem, then use torula yeast), sprinkled on and mixed in the food, is the easiest way to sneak it into a finicky eater's diet.

Most cats, unlike most children, respond enthusiastically to liver. Since it is a fine source of niacin (and all B vitamins), serving B_3 or niacin as a single-meal treat one to three times weekly or adding it to your pet's regular food (being sure that it constitutes no more than 25 percent of the cat's ration) is a good way to ensure niacin sufficiency. The same can be done with any of the foods listed above.

Do not give your cat any of your own niacin supplements. Most supplements come in 50 to 1,000 mg form, much too large a dose for little felines.

B_5
Pantothenic Acid, Calcium Pantothenate, Panthenol

What It Is

- A high-standing member of the water-soluble B complex, cats need daily dietary replacement; particularly important in production of protective antibodies.
- B_5 is necessary for the proper function of adrenal glands (situated outside each kidney and essential for producing cortisone, hormones, and the healthy regulation of virtually all feline metabolic functions).
- It is easily destroyed by canning, heat, food processing techniques and sulfa drugs.
- It is an essential anti-stress vitamin.

Benefits

- Prevents and fights infection by building antibodies.
- Alleviates stress and combats effects of toxins.
- Aids in providing protection and relief from allergies.
- Helps in healing wounds.
- Minimizes adverse side effects of antibiotics.
- Aids in normal functioning of the stomach and intestines.
- Useful in treating sadness.

How Much Is Needed?

The recommended minimum daily allowance is 0.5–1.5 mg for an average, healthy cat. (More is required during illness and stress periods.) Bee pollen, torula and brewer's yeast are full of B_5.

Sources

Liver, kidney, egg yolk (no uncooked whites), wheat germ, bran, chicken, and green vegetables.

Deficiency Symptoms and Diseases

Weight loss, fatty liver disease, and susceptibility to allergies.

Advice

Vitamins B_5, B_6, and B_9 (otherwise known as pantothenic acid, pyridoxine, and folic acid) are the SWAT team protectors of your cat's immune system. Essential contributors to antibody production, these three Bs should be included in your pet's daily diet. (They work better together than alone.)

If you're planning on spaying or neutering your cat, increasing the amount of vitamin B_5, and, of course, B_6 and B_9 in the animal's diet before and after the operation can prevent adverse stress reactions and aid in a speedy recovery. If you are planning a vacation away from your cat—or if your cat is grieving from a loss—B_5 and the other B vitamins are a must.

A cat that's prone to, or suffers from, allergies often has inadequate pantothenic acid and vitamin C production. This can and should be rectified through improved diet or vitamin supplementation. (See cautions for supplementing vitamin C below.)

B_6
Pyridoxine

What It Is

- B_6 is a superstar in the water-soluble B complex, though equally excretable and requiring daily replenishment.
- This is essential for the proper metabolization of a cat's ingested protein and fat, as well as for effective absorption of vitamin B_{12} (cobalamin) and many other nutrients.
- It is indispensable for the production of healthy red blood cells and antibodies.
- It is easily destroyed by long storage, food processing techniques, canning, sterilization, cooking, and water.

Benefits

- Aids in optimal assimilation of protein and fat.
- Fortifies the immune system (particularly when accompanied by pantothenic and folic acids).
- Improves behavior by preventing many nervous disorders.
- Helps in alleviating skin problems.
- Enables proper utilization of essential minerals.
- Useful in treating sadness.
- Required for the nervous system.

How Much Is Needed?

The recommended minimum daily allowance is 0.2–1.5 mg for an average, healthy cat. (More is required during lactation, illness, and stress and growth periods.)

Sources

Brewer's yeast, torula yeast, wheat germ, wheat bran, organ meats (liver, kidney, heart), beef, egg yolk (no uncooked whites), cantaloupe, bee pollen, peas, and avocado.

Deficiency Symptoms and Diseases

Weight loss, inhibited growth, anemia, kidney disease, convulsions, dry or crusting skin, and nervousness.

Advice

Few vitamins are more important for high-protein consumers than B_6. Because cats rank among the highest protein consumers, the need for ample amounts of this vitamin is unquestionable. Since this vitamin is destroyed easily by storage and food processing, I'd suggest that if you're currently feeding your pet generic or low-quality food, you should definitely get some quality pyridoxine into the cat's diet, pronto!

You'll find, once again, that brewer's yeast or torula yeast covers a lot of bases: it's inexpensive, contains all the necessary B vitamins (which, when working synergistically, are much more effective), and is easily made palatable when mixed with your cat's regular fare. Unfortunately, brewer's yeast also contains about 0.17 percent magnesium, and is, therefore, not recommended for cats with FLUTD problems, so use torula instead.

If your cat is being treated with drugs for arthritis or is on an antidepressant, ask your veterinarian if the medication contains Penicillamine. If it does, your pet needs extra vitamin B_6. (Depending upon the treatment, you might want to ask your veterinarian about a professional vitamin supplement.)

CAUTION: Vitamin B_6 can reduce a diabetic cat's need for insulin. To avoid a low blood sugar reaction, consult your veterinarian before making any dietary changes.

B_9
Folic Acid, Folacin, Vitamin M

What It Is

- Yet another water-soluble member of the B complex, B_9 is essential to the healthy development of all parts of a cat's body.
- This is necessary for the effectiveness of other stress-fighting and antibody-building B vitamins. (If not present, effectiveness of other B vitamins is decreased.)
- B_9 is needed for the utilization of amino acids and the formation of red blood cells.
- It can be destroyed by food processing, heat, water, sunlight, sulfa drugs, and storage at room temperatures for extended periods.

Benefits

- Helps maintain a powerful immune system.
- Aids in protecting against intestinal parasites and food poisoning.
- Promotes growth and health of the fetus.
- Improves lactation.
- Stimulates the appetite.

How Much Is Needed?

Though no official minimum daily allowance has been set, 10–25 mg is suggested for an average, healthy cat. (More is required during pregnancy, lactation, stress, and antibiotic treatment.)

Sources

Brewer's yeast, torula yeast, organ meats (liver, kidney, heart), egg yolk (no uncooked whites), cantaloupe, and dark green, leafy vegetables.

Deficiency Symptoms and Diseases

Anemia and weight loss. In kittens: impaired growth.

Advice

A good B complex will give your cat a sufficient amount of folic acid, as it is only required in minute amounts. If your pet is ill or fighting an illness, more folic acid is required, but unless a special supplement is advised by your veterinarian, I'd suggest simply augmenting your cat's diet with any of the multiple B complex foods listed above. Keep the 25 percent rule in mind: by changing only one quarter of your cat's regular meal, you're more likely to enhance the animal's health and less likely to incur feline wrath.

If your cat is pregnant, lactating or on antibiotics, an increase in folic acid is recommended. Since, at times like these, the last thing you want is to take a chance on your cat's rejecting food (which some finicky eaters will do if there's the least alteration in diet), I'd suggest asking your veterinarian for a supplement.

B_{12}
Cobalamin

What It Is

- B_{12} is a water-soluble member of the B complex that, like folic acid, is quite effective in small doses and very necessary.
- It is the only vitamin that also contains essential mineral elements.
- On commercial food labels, it is often listed as the additive cobalamin concentrate or cyanocobalamin.
- Its absorption can be impaired by a poorly functioning thyroid gland.
- It is most effective when accompanied by foods containing all the B complex vitamins, as well as vitamins A, E, and C. Additionally, it must combine with calcium during absorption to be of benefit to the animal's body.
- It is found only in animal sources, not plants or vegetables.

Benefits

- Improves the immune system and prevents anemia.
- Aids in effective metabolization of protein, fat and carbohydrates.
- Alleviates behavior problems by promoting a healthy nervous system.
- Promotes growth and increases appetite in kittens and young cats.
- Helps in many intestinal tract problems.

How Much Is Needed?

No standard daily allowance has been established for cats, but a minimum of 5 mg is recommended.

Sources

Liver and other animal organ meats, beef, pork, cheese, and egg yolk (no uncooked whites).

Deficiency Symptoms and Diseases

Anemia, impaired growth, susceptibility to infection, abnormal gait, and digestive problems.

Advice

Like folic acid, a little vitamin B_{12} goes a long way. In fact, it works best with folic acid (along with the rest of the B complex vitamins and vitamins A, E, and C) and can be a real energizer for lethargic cats.

An imbalanced diet—one that's low in vitamin B_1 and high in folic acid (which I've seen when owners decide they want their cats to become vegetarians)—can not only cause a vitamin B_{12} deficiency, but can also hide it for quite a while from all but the most extensive (and expensive) medical tests.

Steer clear of all store-bought B_{12} supplements, unless they are prescribed by your veterinarian.

BIOTIN
Vitamin H, Coenzyme R

What It Is

- This is a water-soluble member of the B complex that is required by cats in small amounts and aids in synthesis of vitamin C.
- This is necessary for effective metabolism of protein, fat and carbohydrates.
- Avidin (a protein found in raw egg whites) can prevent absorption of biotin and, therefore, its usefulness in the body.
- Biotin works synergistically with riboflavin, niacin, pyridoxine and vitamin A in keeping a cat's skin and coat healthy.
- Food processing techniques, water, sulfa drugs, and raw egg whites can destroy its effectiveness.
- It can be made in the intestines by bacteria.

Benefits

- Helps prevent hair loss, dermatitis, and other skin conditions.
- Aids in maintaining proper thyroid and adrenal gland function.
- Promotes a healthy nervous system.
- Assists in providing optimal metabolization of food.

How Much Is Needed?

The recommended minimum daily allowance is 15 mg for an average, healthy cat.

Sources

Torula yeast, brewer's yeast, egg yolk (no uncooked whites), beef liver, kidney, unpolished rice (ground), and milk.

Deficiency Symptoms and Diseases

Runny eyes, nasal discharge, loss of appetite (anorexia), severe weight loss, scaly patches on the face, and bloody diarrhea.

Advice

Don't give your cat raw egg whites. Use just the yolk, or cook the egg. This will prevent a lot of nutritional problems and allow your cat to benefit from the biotin content in the meals you're feeding.

Your cat's need for biotin is increased during antibiotic or sulfa drug therapy, but a prepared supplement is rarely necessary. Good B complex additions to the diet will usually provide a sufficient amount of this nutrient. (If the treatment is for an extended period of time, and your pet is displaying signs of deficiency, consult your vet for a supplement.) A healthy bacterial flora in your cat's intestine is very important. There are two types of friendly bacteria that will help produce biotin. Yogurt contains both of them: acidophillus and bifida.

CHOLINE & INOSITOL

What It Is

- These are water-soluble members of the B complex vitamins that work together in metabolizing fats and cholesterol for effective utilization.
- Lipotropics (fat emulsifiers) help transport fat. They help excess fat move out of the liver and distribute it throughout the body. They form lecithin.

Benefits

- Helps the liver eliminate poisons and drugs from the body.
- Enhances nerve impulse transmission and improves memory.
- Modifies excitability and produces a calming effect.

How Much Is Needed?

For an average, healthy cat, the recommended minimum daily allowance of choline is 50 to 100 mg and 10–25 mg of inositol.

Sources

Egg yolk (no uncooked whites), organ meats, wheat germ, brewer's yeast, green, leafy vegetables, and cantaloupe.

Deficiency Symptoms and Diseases

Possibly fatty liver disease, rough, scaly skin (eczema), and nervousness.

Advice

Since most foods containing B complex vitamins also contain choline and inositol, there is no need for special or additional supplementation. I say this on the assumption that by now you realize how important B complex vitamins are to a cat's well-being. (If you don't, go back and reread this chapter.)

Perhaps the one exception to choline and inositol supplementation might be the necessity to maximize your cat's vitamin E intake, and you don't want to risk overdosing your pet. Choline and inositol are safe, natural and effective for vitamin E absorption.

CAUTION: Choline is inadvisable for cats with liver disease.

VITAMIN C
Ascorbic Acid, Cevitamic Acid

What It Is

- This is a water-soluble vitamin that cats can synthesize in their bodies (in the liver), but in amounts too small to provide significant health benefits or immune protection.
- Excreted in urine, it is used up rapidly during periods of stress,

growth and illness, and must be replaced through dietary sources.
- Cooking, heat, light, water, exposure to air and certain medications destroy vitamin C.
- It is essential in forming collagen (the primary constituent of connective tissue, bone, and cartilage), and necessary for growth and repair of a cat's teeth, gums, bones, blood vessels, and tissue cells.
- It is needed for the animal's proper absorption of iron.
- On food labels, it often appears as the additive ascorbic acid or sodium ascorbate.

Benefits

- Improves the immune system and aids in preventing many types of viral and bacterial infections.
- Alleviates allergies (can inhibit release of histamine).
- Provides protection from toxins (either in food or in the environment).
- Helps build strong teeth, gums and limbs, and retards deterioration of them as the animal ages.
- Aids in preventing cystitis and feline urinary problems.
- Helps counteract side effects of steroids (which are often used to reduce itching or increase appetite in animals) that interfere with collagen formation.
- Can relieve joint pain.
- Helps prevent cancer and feline leukemia.
- Helps in treatment of respiratory and liver diseases.
- Speeds up healing after surgery.
- An absolute essential for a feline AIDS or leukemia cat!

How Much Is Needed?

No minimum daily allowance has yet been established for cats, since they are capable of manufacturing the vitamin—not, however, in the amount needed for either disease prevention or general well-being. However, 50–100 mg is advised. (During illness, vitamin C synthesis is impaired and 100–500 mg daily is recommended.)

Sources

Tomato juice, cantaloupe, green, leafy vegetables, rhubarb, asparagus, bee pollen, green peas, and liver.

Deficiency Symptoms and Diseases

Inflammation of the gums (gingivitis), joint and muscle pain, fatigue, and brittle bones (all possible symptoms of subclinical scurvy).

Advice

For an effective immune system, cats definitely need more vitamin C than the small amount their bodies produce. This is especially true for indoor cats. Outdoor cats can supplement their supply of vitamin C by hunting or eating their prey, which, if it's a mouse, has this vitamin in large supply. These outdoor hunters might not devour all of what they kill, but they'll almost always eat the liver (where ascorbic acid is made), the adrenal glands (where it is stored), and some muscle tissue (which also contains the vitamin).

Stress of any kind (illness, a new pet in the home, travel, and so on) calls for more vitamin C than most cats can produce to combat the stress successfully. This lowers their resistance, making them more vulnerable to infections (viral and bacterial) and to disease, in effect leaving them with an immune system that's not even worth its name.

Most cat foods are not fortified with vitamin C, despite increasing evidence that this vitamin is invaluable to feline well-being, so it's a good idea to supplement your pet's diet. Though natural vitamin C is found primarily in fruits and vegetables (not, admittedly, feline favorites), many cats do enjoy the taste of tomato juice. (Don't knock it if your cat hasn't tried it.) Just a little added to your pet's food each day may help keep urine acidic and aid in preventing cystitis and other common urinary ailments.

Feline vitamin C supplements are available at pet stores or can be obtained from your veterinarian. Always follow the directions on

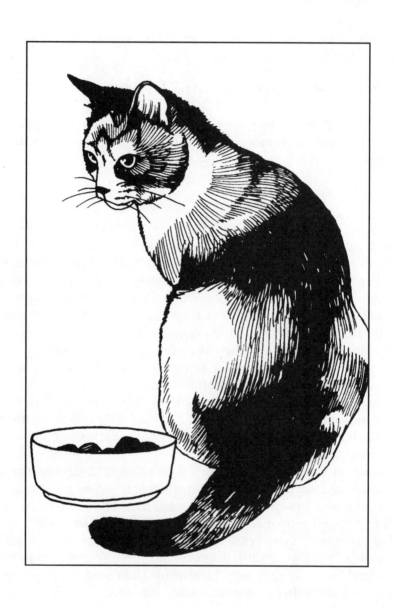

the label. (Too much vitamin C can cause diarrhea, among other unpleasant side effects.)

IMPORTANT: Before starting any supplement regimen, check with your veterinarian.

Vitamin C supplement is the same for humans and cats. Most vitamin C is acidic, so your cat won't like the powder, and you have to be careful when giving it vitamin C pills because the pills can burn the esophagus.

I prefer to give Ester C powder. It is a neutral, very effective vitamin C with almost no taste. Simply put it into a salt shaker and sprinkle onto the food. When Ester C is combined with bioflavanoids it makes it even better. By the way, city cats and cats who live with smokers need extra vitamin C.

VITAMIN D

The "Sunshine Vitamin," Calciferol, Ergosterol

What It Is

- This is a fat-soluble vitamin that cats obtain primarily from sunlight. (Ultraviolet rays, acting on the animal's skin oils, produce the vitamin, which is then absorbed into the body.)
- When obtained through food (essentially fish oils), it is absorbed with fats through the intestinal walls.
- It can be stored in the body and does not require daily replenishment. (An oversupply can cause hypervitaminosis D: an uneven distribution of calcium in the bones, abnormal teeth, a dangerous hardening of soft tissue in lungs, kidneys, heart, and blood vessels.)
- On food labels it is often listed as the additive calciferol, ergocalciferol, or cholecalciferol.
- It is necessary for the proper utilization of calcium and phosphorus.

Benefits

- Promotes strong bones and teeth.

How Much Is Needed?

The recommended minimum daily allowance is 50–100 IU for an average, healthy cat.

Sources

Sunlight, egg yolk (no uncooked whites), fish oils, liver, and fish.

Deficiency Symptoms and Diseases

Malformation of bones and teeth and weak muscles and joints (rickets).

Advice

Beware of supplementing this vitamin unless you've been instructed to do so by your veterinarian. Though it's true that an insufficient supply of vitamin D can impede your cat's absorption of needed calcium, the chances of feline vitamin D deficiency are rare.

Do not use cod liver oil (or any other fish oil) as a routine daily dietary supplement. If you're under the impression that doing this is the way to improve your cat's coat or strengthen bones and teeth, you're wrong. Moreover, you're seriously endangering your pet's health by inviting hypervitaminosis D.

VITAMIN E
Tocopherol

What It Is

- This is a fat-soluble vitamin that, unlike some others (A, D, and K), is stored only for a relatively short time in the body.
- It is an important antioxidant, preventing oxidation of fat compounds, vitamin A, selenium, some vitamin C and other nutrients.

- Vitamin E can be destroyed by food processing, extremes in temperature, iron, chlorine, and mineral oil.
- It often appears on food labels as the additive alpha tocopherol acetate, alpha tocopherol concentrate, or alpha tocopherol acid succinate.

Benefits

- Strengthens the immune system.
- Provides protection against environmental pollutants and toxins.
- Retards cellular aging, boosts endurance, and promotes rejuvenative behavior.
- Aids in prevention of steatitis (caused by all-fish diets).
- Helps in curing skin problems.
- Enhances fertility.
- Enables other nutrients to function more effectively.

How Much Is Needed?

The recommended minimum daily allowance is 5–15 IU for an average, healthy cat. (More is needed when the cat's diet is high in polyunsaturated fats, found in canned tuna fish.)

Sources

Wheat germ, broccoli, spinach, egg yolk (no uncooked whites), enriched flour, and liver.

Deficiency Symptoms and Diseases

A combination of fatigue, loss of appetite, and generalized soreness and fever due to inflammation of body fat (steatitis). It creates sores on the body.

Advice

If you live in a city, it's important to include ample vitamin E in your cat's diet. Vitamin E works with beta-carotene and vitamin C as an antioxidant, protecting your pet from the harmful effects of pollutants. These three vitamins, which make each other more effective, also maximize cellular membrane strength, keeping your cat's stored fat safe from oxidation. They also keep fat prepared to help ward off invasion by unwanted bacteria and viruses.

The best prevention against vitamin E deficiency is to keep your cat away from raw fish, cat foods with red tuna meat and your own canned tuna fish. If your cat is a fish freak and refuses to change, mix some wheat germ (one-half to one teaspoon) into your pet's daily meals. This can help counteract the possibility that your cat will develop steatitis.

Many commercial cat vitamin and mineral supplements contain insufficient amounts of vitamin E. If your cat is showing signs of steatitis (for example, yowls when you stroke its back, doesn't move around much), eliminate fish and fish-based food from the diet and get in touch with your veterinarian immediately.

VITAMIN K
Menadione

What It Is

- This is a fat-soluble vitamin that a cat can form in the intestines.
- It is necessary in forming the blood-clotting substance prothrombin.
- Vitamin K can be depleted by X rays, radiation, mineral oil and certain sulfa medicines used to treat urinary tract infections.
- It often appears on food labels as the additive phytonadione.

Benefits

- Aids in preventing internal bleeding and hemorrhages.
- Promotes effective blood clotting.

How Much Is Needed?

There is no recommended daily allowance since cats manufacture their own vitamin K, which is normally sufficient.

Sources

Egg yolk (no uncooked whites), yogurt, leafy, green vegetables, alfalfa sprouts, and liver.

Deficiency Symptoms and Diseases

Poor blood clotting (hypoprothrombonemia).

Advice

Cats rarely develop a vitamin K deficiency, except, perhaps, if they are being overdosed with mineral oil or are on an extended sulfur medication program or have kidney disease. Yogurt or alfalfa sprouts added to your pet's diet are healthy, safe, and nutritious preventives.

Excessive bloody diarrhea could indicate an insufficiency of vitamin K, but this should be checked out immediately by your veterinarian.

If you are taking an anticoagulant medication such as Coumadin (warfarin), keep it out of an inquisitive cat's reach. Ingestion of warfarin (which is also in rat poisons) can dangerously deplete your pet of vitamin K and cause abnormal bleeding.

CAUTION: If your cat is being treated with heparin, an anticoagulant occasionally used in the treatment of DIC (disseminated intravascular coagulation), be aware that even natural foods containing vitamin K can reverse the drug's effect.

MINERALS

Without minerals, vitamins are virtually useless, because they can not be assimilated and though cats can synthesize some vitamins in their bodies, they can not manufacture a single mineral.

CALCIUM

What It Is

- Calcium is the mineral that, along with phosphorus, is most required in a cat's diet.
- It must exist in the diet with approximately equal quantities of phosphorus (a calcium/phosphorus ratio of 1:1) to function properly and to maintain strong teeth and bones, and a healthy nervous system.
- For effective absorption and utilization of calcium, vitamin D must be present.

Benefits

- Promotes growth and maintenance of strong bones and teeth.
- Improves behavior by keeping the nervous system functioning properly.
- Aids in blood clotting.

How Much Is Needed?

The recommended minimum daily allowance is 200–400 mg for an average, healthy cat. (More is required during pregnancy, lactation, and kitten growth periods.)

Sources

Milk and milk products, cheese, sardines, and green vegetables.

Deficiency Symptoms and Diseases

Decrease in bone density, limping, aversion to activity and movement, and spontaneous fractures (osteoporosis). In nursing queens: trembling and rigidity (eclampsia). In kittens: swollen tender joints, arched back, and stiff legs (rickets).

Advice

Avoid feeding your cat an all-meat diet and you'll avoid many problems. Meat-rich diets can cause a deficiency in calcium. Because meat has about fifteen times more phosphorus than calcium (organ meats, such as heart, liver, and kidney, have almost thirty to fifty times as much), the imbalance can cause your pet serious harm (see deficiency symptoms above).

Obviously, prevention is the best cure; but if it's too late for that, I'd suggest increasing the calcium in your cat's diet. Supplements are available in several forms, so ask your veterinarian about the right type and dosage for your pet. (If your cat likes ricotta cheese, one quarter cup will supply 167 mg of additional calcium.) Be patient; deficiencies are not reversed overnight.

Don't attempt to overload your cat with calcium. This can result in other bone abnormalities, as well as decrease absorption, and cause possible deficiencies of zinc, iron, iodine, and phosphorus.

It's important to remember that even though vitamin D is necessary for calcium absorption, an existing calcium deficiency, or calcium/phosphorous imbalance, can be worsened by adding more vitamin D to the diet.

Pregnant or nursing cats don't need, and should not have, additional calcium; they should eat kitten food which has all they need. If you absolutely must add calcium, then do so in a natural form (cottage cheese, lactose-free milk).

COBALT

What It Is

- Cobalt is essentially a part of vitamin B_{12} (cobalamin) that's needed for the manufacturing of red blood cells.

Benefits

- Helps prevent anemia.

How Much Is Needed?

The recommended minimum daily allowance is .016–0.2 mg for an average, healthy cat.

Sources

Meat, kidney, liver, milk, oysters, and clams.

Deficiency Symptoms and Diseases

Same as for vitamin B_{12}.

Advice

Cobalt is only required when vitamin B_{12} is deficient. Since strict vegetarians are the only group I know prone to B_{12} deficiency, and I know of no cats that are strict vegetarians, I feel confident in telling you not to worry about your pet's cobalt intake.

COPPER

What It Is

- This mineral is necessary for converting the iron in your cat's body into hemoglobin (the iron-containing pigment in red blood cells that carry oxygen from the lungs to the tissues).

- Copper is important for the effective utilization of vitamin C.
- It is often listed on food labels as the additive copper gluconate or cupric sulfate.

Benefits

- Increases energy and alertness by aiding effective iron absorption.

How Much Is Needed?

The recommended minimum daily allowance is 0.02 mg for an average, healthy cat.

Sources

Beef, liver, and peas.

Deficiency Symptoms and Diseases

Rare.

Advice

Relax. Your pet is getting adequate amounts of copper through meats and other animal products that are staples in cat diets.

IODINE

What It Is

- A particularly vital mineral for cats, it affects the function of the thyroid gland, which controls metabolism.
- Paradoxically, an undersupply can cause either hypothyroidism or hyperthyroidism (see deficiency symptoms below).
- It is contained in many prepared foods in the form of iodized salt.

Benefits

- Promotes growth and alertness.
- Aids in weight control by burning excess fat.
- Helps prevent and remedy both hypothyroidism and hyper-thyroidism.

How Much Is Needed?

The recommended minimum daily allowance is 0.01–0.02 mg for an average, healthy cat.

Sources

Seafood (for example, shrimp or scallops), vegetables grown in iodine-rich soil, and kelp.

Deficiency Symptoms and Diseases

Lethargy, slow mental reaction, unexplainable weight gain (hypothyroidism), bulging eyeballs, nervous irritability, ravenous appetite, emaciation, and enlarged thyroid gland (goiter or hyper-thyroidism).

Advice

Virtually all cat foods contain iodized salt, so the chances of your pet developing a specific iodine-related deficiency is rare. Other malfunctions of the thyroid gland can cause the conditions I've mentioned above and should be diagnosed and treated only by a veterinarian.

IRON

What It Is

- Iron is vital to forming red blood corpuscles (hemoglobin), which transport oxygen to body tissues.
- It is important for the proper metabolization of B vitamins.
- It is easily available and readily utilized from meat products as long as the cat has an adequate supply of copper, cobalt, manganese, and vitamin C.

Benefits

- Improves the immune system and resistance to disease.
- Aids growth.
- Reduces absorption of lead and helps prevent its harmful effects.
- Cures or prevents an unlikely occurrence of iron-deficient anemia.

How Much Is Needed?

The recommended minimum daily allowance is 5 mg for an average, healthy cat.

Sources

Liver, kidney, heart, farina, red meat, egg yolk (no uncooked whites), asparagus, oatmeal, bran, lettuce, beets, tomatoes, and cornmeal.

Deficiency Symptoms and Diseases

Impaired growth and lethargy (iron-deficient animals).

Advice

If you think feeding milk instead of cat food is spoiling your pet, you're underestimating the impact of your action: you're ruining the animal's health! Cow's milk contains only a very small amount of iron. And unless the milk is mixed with an iron-rich cereal, the nutritional benefits, especially as far as promoting growth and preventing anemia, are zero.

Iron supplements to a balanced diet are rarely needed.

Pet tinic is an excellent (veterinary only) tonic for anemic, run-down cats. Ask your veterinarian about it.

MAGNESIUM

What It Is

- This mineral is important for the proper metabolism and usefulness of vitamins C, E, and B complex, calcium, phosphorus, sodium, and potassium.
- It is used to convert blood sugar into energy.
- It is essential for nerve and muscle function.
- Magnesium is the prime, oversupplied ash culprit in FLUTD.
- It is often listed on food labels as magnesium phosphate or magnesium sulfate.

Benefits

- Helps regulate body temperature and improve the cardiovascular system.
- Aids in modifying agitated behavior by working with calcium as a natural tranquilizer.
- Helps with constipation.

How Much Is Needed?

The recommended minimum daily allowance is 4–8 mg for an average, healthy cat.

Sources

Shrimp, ground nuts, sardines, breast of chicken, and tuna.

Deficiency Symptoms and Diseases

Rare.

Advice

Watch out for oversupplying your pet with magnesium. Most foods that cats eat supply much more magnesium than is needed, and it's the magnesium in ash (not ash alone) that primarily causes and aggravates FLUTD and other urinary ailments. In fact, I recommend avoiding any dry food that contains more than 0.1 percent magnesium.

If your cat has urinary problems, do not use a daily multi-vitamin-mineral supplement without a veterinarian's approval. Most of these contain at least seven or more milligrams of magnesium.

MANGANESE

What It Is

- This is an important mineral for good bone growth and structure.
- It is necessary for a cat's proper utilization of biotin, vitamins B_1, C, and E, and fat metabolism.
- It aids in forming the principal hormone of the thyroid gland (thyroxine).

Benefits

- Improves agility and alertness.
- Helps alleviate behavior problems by reducing nervousness.

How Much Is Needed?

The recommended minimum daily allowance is 0.2 mg for an average, healthy cat.

Sources

Egg yolk (no uncooked whites), beets, whole-grain cereals, leafy, green vegetables, and peas.

Deficiency Symptoms and Diseases

Rare.

Advice

Manganese is ample in most cat diets, so you don't have to worry about getting extra amounts into your pet's meals. Though this mineral is included in most commercial cat supplements, which advise one-half to one tablet per day, the chance of any sort of toxicity is rare.

If you're feeding your cat a diet with very high amounts of calcium and phosphorus (see listings above and below), be aware that it could inhibit the absorption of manganese.

Note: Do not confuse manganese with magnesium.

PHOSPHOROUS

What It Is

- Phosphorous is the mineral that works with calcium and is, therefore, indispensable in your cat's diet.
- It should exist in a cat's diet with approximately equal quantities of calcium to function properly in maintaining strong bones and teeth and a healthy nervous system (vitamin D is also necessary for effective utilization of calcium).
- Excessive amounts can result in calcium deficiency.
- It's found in many commercial foods, where it is listed as the additive calcium phytosphate, sodium phosphate or sodium pyrophosphate.
- It can be rendered ineffective by too much iron or magnesium.

Benefits

- Increases energy by aiding metabolization of fats and starches.
- Helps healing of bone and other injuries.
- Promotes healthier gums, teeth, and growth.

How Much Is Needed?

The recommended minimum daily allowance is 150–400 mg for an average, healthy cat.

Sources

Meat, egg yolk (no uncooked whites), fish (cooked), and whole grains.

Deficiency Symptoms and Diseases

Rare.

Advice

Phosphorus is plentiful in animal protein, so deficiencies are rare. Unfortunately, excesses are not. It's important to always keep the calcium/phosphorus ratio in mind. It's calcium/phosphorus 0.9:1 to 1.1:1.

When you feed a balanced diet, your cat will get all the benefits and none of the risks of phosphorus deficiency. (Those risks, by the way, can add up to problems if your pet is hooked on a single food with an inverse calcium/phosphorus ratio.) I feel strongly that all cats should be fed at least two different foods to prevent unhealthy addictions.

POTASSIUM

What It Is

- Working with sodium, this mineral regulates a cat's heart rhythms and water balance, and enables nerve impulses to be carried effectively to and from the brain.
- It is a nutrient that can be depleted by diarrhea, excessive sugar, diuretic medicines, severe stress or kidney disease.
- On commercial foods it is often listed as one of the following additives: potassium chloride, potassium glycerophosphate, or potassium iodide.

Benefits

- Helps improve mental and muscular reflexes.
- Aids in allergy treatments and elimination of body wastes.

How Much Is Needed?

The recommended minimum daily allowance is 50–100 mg for an average, healthy cat.

Sources

Beef, poultry, fish, cantaloupe, tomatoes, green, leafy vegetables, bananas, cereals, and garlic.

Deficiency Symptoms and Diseases

Can be caused by excessive diarrhea, use of certain diuretic medication, or kidney disease.

Advice

Unless your cat is on some sort of diuretic medication or has kidney disease (in which case, you should ask your veterinarian about what foods or supplements ought to be included in the animal's diet), or unless you're feeding your cat excessive amounts of sugary treats, don't worry about your pet getting enough potassium.

SODIUM

What It Is

- Works with potassium to regulate fluid balance, muscle contraction, and nerve stimulation.
- Helps keep calcium and other vital minerals soluble (and, therefore, usable) in blood.
- In a word: salt!

Benefits

- Helps keep reflexes at optimal performance.
- Aids in preventing heat prostration.
- Regulates blood pressure.

How Much Is Needed?

The recommended daily allowance is not to exceed 15% of the diet of the average, healthy cat.

Sources

Salt (ample in all commercial cat food), shellfish, kidney, beets, bacon, and grains.

Deficiency Symptoms and Diseases

Possible weight and fur loss and dry skin. (Deficiency of sodium chloride is rare, except when heat or extreme exercise causes excessive loss of water and salt.)

Advice

Trust me on this one: your cat is getting enough dietary sodium if you are feeding him any commercial brand of cat food.

Salt (not in excess, of course) is good for cats, because it makes them want to drink water—and water is essential, particularly for dry-food eaters and older cats. Cats with heart disease, high blood pressure, or kidney disease may need a special, low-sodium diet, available from your family veterinarian.

ZINC

What It Is

- A top-notch major mineral, zinc is necessary for protein synthesis, development of reproductive organs, contractibility of muscles and tissue reconstruction.
- It is destroyed by food processing.
- In commercial foods, it is often listed as the additive zinc oxide or zinc sulfate.

Benefits

- Aids in wound healing: burns, lacerations, flea bites and skin abrasions.
- Helps promote growth and mental alertness.
- Aids in removing toxins from the body and protecting against cancer.
- Helps build a healthy immune system.

How Much Is Needed?

The recommended minimum daily allowance is 0.25–0.5 mg for an average, healthy cat.

Sources

Lamb, pork, beef, egg yolk (no uncooked whites), wheat germ, brewer's yeast, and torula yeast.

Deficiency Symptoms and Diseases

Retarded growth, weight loss, vomiting, and conjunctivitis.

Advice

If your cat's diet is high in soy meal (check labels), more zinc is probably necessary in the animal's diet.

Zinc functions best when your cat gets adequate amounts of calcium, phosphorus, and vitamin A. Zinc is useful and works well with antioxidants such as vitamin E, selenium, and beta-carotene.

HERBS AND OTHER THINGS

ACIDOPHILUS

What It Is

Sour milk and yogurt are known for their acidophilus content, which works by assisting in the digestion of proteins and keeps the right balance of good and bad bacteria. It's almost tasteless.

Benefits

- Helpful in control of diarrhea, especially in kittens and strays.
- Helps to keep the intestinal cells healthy.

How Much Is Needed?

500,000 to 1 million units in the food daily. It can be bought in powder form.

Sources

Best high-quality acidophilus source for your cat:
- Yogurt for cats under 1 year of age.
- Bene Bac manufactured by Pet Ag.
- Acidophilus powder for humans.

ALOE VERA

What It Is

- A plant used for over 4,000 years for its various medicinal properties.
- There are over 200 different types throughout the world.

Benefits

- It's known as a skin healer; moisturizer for use on sores.
- Used for regularity—an excellent laxative for constipated cats.

How Much Is Needed?

Externally, just rub it on the wound. You can also use it on mouth ulcers.

As a laxative, use either the tablet or the liquid-gel cap. Put 10 mg of aloe vera concentrate, or approximately 1/4 to 1/2 teaspoon into your cat's food—look at the results that evening and the next morning. You will probably alter the dosage depending on your cat's metabolism.

If you give too much, you may get diarrhea.

Sources

Health food stores will give you a great choice—select the ones that don't have much of a taste.

ALFALFA

What It Is

- One of the richest mineral foods, because of its deep roots.
- Among the many elements it contains: calcium, magnesium, phosphorous, potassium, and vitamins.

Benefits

- Providing your cat isn't having FLUTD problems, it's a great mineral supplement.
- Can provide relief from pain and stiffness due to aging and/or arthritis.

How Much Is Needed?

Alfalfa has a minty taste and may be difficult to give to your cat.

I suggest putting fresh ground alfalfa into a salt shaker and adding one shake at a time.

Don't exceed 4 shakes.

1/8–1/4 tablet (human) daily. Don't break it up into the food because your cat probably won't eat it. If you put some butter on the tablet, it will be easier to pill your cat.

Sources

Best high-quality alfalfa source for your cat:
- Health food stores and mail-order herbal catalogues.
- Animals' Apawthecary carries better-tasting formulas (1-800-822-9609).

BEE POLLEN

What It Is

- A fine powderlike material made by the anthers of flowering plants and gathered by the bee.
- Claimed to be one of the oldest complete food in the world.
- Has a sweet/sour taste that cats generally like.

Benefits

- A "natural" antiobiotic.
- Promotes healthy gums and immune system.
- Useful in allergies.

How Much Is Needed?

As a preventative, a salt shaker on each meal, otherwise 1/8 teaspoon twice daily. Not to be used if your cat is a diabetic.

Sources

Health food stores.

Advice

I recommend bee pollen as THE daily supplement of choice. All the proteins, fats, vitamins, minerals, etc., have been balanced by nature—and won't interfere with the food you are feeding.

I have combined this fabulous all around preventative with vegetable enzymes in a product called Dr. Jane® Beezyme. The natural enzymes assure more digestion of your cat's food and complete absorption of the bee pollen!

CHAMOMILE

What It Is

- "Anthemis nobilis,"an herb also called Whig plant. It has beneficial medicinal properties.

Benefits

- Helpful in diarrhea or upset stomach.
- The tea can be made into an eye wash for irritated eyes.
- Can have calming effects.

How Much Is Needed?

As a tincture: (ask for one without alcohol), 1–3 drops in the water dish, or directly into your cat's mouth once or twice daily.
As a tea: add 1/8 teaspoon to canned food, or mix with dry food.

Sources

Health food stores, supermarkets, and herbal catalogues.

DANDELION

What It Is

- An herb named "Taraxacum densleonis," also called lion's tooth, white endive.
- It has beneficial medicinal properties.
- Rich with iron,vitamin Bs, sulfur, zinc, and many nutritive salts.

Benefits

- May be useful in weight loss programs.
- Can be a natural diuretic for cats with heart disease (ask your veterinarian).

- Can be useful for cats with anemia or kidney disease.
- Is used after constipation to help move everything out!

How Much Is Needed?

For weight loss, simply chop up fresh dandelion and add it to your cat's food; a little each day until he gets used to its rather bitter taste!

For an aid in anemia, constipation, or heart disease use a tincture: (without alcohol) 2–3 drops in the food daily or in the mouth once daily.

Sources

- Fresh produce stores during the season.
- Health food stores for tinctures.
- Animals' Apawthecary carries better-tasting herbs (1-800-822-9609).

ECHINACEA

What It Is

- An herb named "Echinacea angustifolia" or purple cone flower.
- Very bitter tasting.
- It has beneficial medicinal properties, known as an antibacterial, antiviral herb.

Benefits

- Use it to build up your cat's immune system when it has colds, has just undergone an operation, has a wound or has been exposed to a sick cat.

How Much Is Needed?

As a tincture (without alcohol) 2–3 drops every 4 hours during the first 3 days, decreasing to twice daily.

Do not use this herb for more than 7 days.

Sources

- Health food stores and herbal catalogues.
- Animals' Apawthecary carries better-tasting herbs (1-800-822-9609).

Advice

Echinacea is a great herb for humans, but cats really don't like it. If you are successful in giving it to your cat—congratulations. Don't get me wrong, many people are stubborn enough to succeed and have been pleased with the results. The 7-day limit is one that I put on all herbal remedies with some exceptions. Sometimes a body needs to rest in between remedies, and keep in mind that even natural substances can become toxic!

GARLIC

What It Is

- An herb used for taste and medicinal properties.
- Described as a natural antibiotic/antiparasitic substance.
- Contains potassium, useful for older cats.

Benefits

- Strengthens the immune system.
- Garlic powder sprinkled on food will enhance its flavor.
- Garlic oil helps promote healthy skin and coat.
- Garlic combined with brewer's yeast is said to repel fleas.

How Much Is Needed?

1/8–1/4 chopped, raw garlic.

Sources

- Can be purchased as a gel capsule from grocery or health food stores.
- Supermarkets—whole fresh garlic

Advice

Even though a study done at a major university demonstrated that garlic and brewer's yeast did not repel fleas, I owned a feline boarding kennel and will tell you that the cats on brewer's yeast and garlic had no fleas! It's the type of natural supplement that you can't go wrong with! I suggest its use in senior cats to keep all their organs functioning right! Among its many features, it detoxifies the body, strengthens blood vessels, helps circulation, and helps fight infection.

HOPS

What It Is

- An herb named "Humulus lupulus" is an old-fashioned remedy for nervousness.
- Contains many nutrients, including vitamin B_6, choline and inositol.

Benefits

- The herb of choice for cats with nocturnal behavior.
- Used for cats recovering from trauma—it's a pain killer.

How Much Is Needed?

One dropperful of hops tea before bed, or as much hops tea as you can put into canned food or mix with dry. Sprinkle dry hops onto canned food.

Sources

- Health food stores and herbal catalogues.
- Animals' Apawthecary carries better-tasting herbs (1-800-822-9609).

Advice

Cats tend to be night animals, so let's face it—they like to play at night. If you plan to get to bed by 11, make sure you exercise your cat, feed it, give it warm milk and honey, and if that's still not enough—a dropper of hops tea sweetened with honey will usually calm down the most persistent of cats. It can be combined with chamomile.

Water: The Nutrient You Never Think About

Let me state this briefly, succinctly, and emphatically: cats need water. They can lose almost all of their body fat and protein and still survive; but if they lose more than one-tenth of their body water, they can't survive. (Ironically, they are able to live without water longer than humans, but unrectified dehydration is inevitably fatal for both.)

In areas where there is hard water, cats get extra calcium and magnesium. If your pet has FLUTD, you might consider giving the animal bottled water that doesn't have a high magnesium content.

Always keep fresh water available for your cat. I like to add water to canned food, as much as your cat will tolerate.

Q&A

Veggie Vexation

I'm sure my cat needs more roughage in his diet, because he's often constipated. But how can I get him to eat raw vegetables?

I've found that grating and then marinating them in melted butter or chicken fat works best. Add just a pinch to his food to begin, and I do mean just a pinch. Too much will turn him off immediately. Once he begins accepting it, increase the amount (just slightly) each day until you find you can add 1–3 tablespoons of grated greens, carrots, beets, sprouts (or boiled green beans, broccoli or cauliflower) to his daily diet. Even better, add some brewer's yeast or torula yeast and bran mix to his meals, or if you prefer, add canned pumpkin, just about 1/8–1/4 teaspoon daily. Pumpkin is great for constipation. Also be sure he's eating a highly digestible food and getting ample liquids.

If the constipation continues, consult your veterinarian. More than just a dietary deficiency might be the cause.

Allergy Defense

When we take Mushka, our five-year-old, male Siamese, with us to our country home in the summer, he sneezes, scratches, loses hair and looks terrible. We don't let him outside and we feed him the same food we always do. Do you think this is a stress-psychological reaction or some sort of allergy? And what can we do about it?

As prone to mood swings and unpredictable behavior as Siamese cats are, I suspect that Mushka is allergic to something (dust, mold, airborne spores) in your country home. I suggest supplementing his daily diet with 100–200 mg of vitamin C, a natural antihistamine, for at least a month or two before you plan to leave, and then continue the supplementation while you're there.

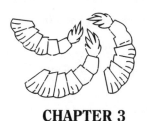

CHAPTER 3

. . . .

Must-Knows
for Mealtimes

. . . .

The Wrong Way to Feed a Feline

*Don't feed your cat the way you would feed a dog
or a human being.*

Probably the biggest mistake people make about feeding is thinking that because both cats and dogs have paws and fur and often live as pets in the same household, their care and diet are the same. Wrong!

- Adult cats need almost five times more protein than do adult dogs.
- Cats require the amino acid taurine (which dogs do not) and must have it in their daily diet. (See "Protein" in chapter 2.)
- Cats need a daily intake of more B vitamins than dogs.
- Dog food is nutritionally deficient for cats!

A second mistake is the belief that what's good for people must be good or better for cats. Wrong!

- Canned tuna, which is fine for people, can kill a cat if fed as a daily diet.
- Cats have uniquely high nutritional needs for meeting their daily energy (k-cal or calorie) requirements with quality, high-

73

BF protein. (See chapter 2 for other "Differences That Make the Difference.")

Counting Your Cat's Calories

When filling your cat's calorie requirements, do it with calories that count nutritionally.

It's extremely important to remember that quality protein—protein that is going to supply the proper amount of amino acids—is vital to your cat's health. A nutritious diet for an adult cat should contain a minimum of 30 percent of its calories from quality protein and a minimum of 20 to 40 percent from the right fats. (See Chapter 2.)

••••••••••••••••••••••••••••••

Quick Converter

1 gram protein	= 4 calories
1 gram carbohydrate	= 4 calories
1 gram fat	= 9 calories

••••••••••••••••••••••••••••••

Basic Calorie Needs for Cats

Age	Daily Requirement per Pound of Body Weight	Approximate Amount Needed Daily
Newborn	190	50
1–5 weeks	125	125
5–10 weeks	100	200
10–20 weeks	65	290
20–30 weeks	50	325
Adult tom	40	400
Adult queen (pregnant)	50	375
Adult queen (lactating)	125	690
Adult male (neutered)	40	360
Adult female (spayed)	40	220

There is a limit to how much—or how little—will satisfy your cat at mealtime. Therefore, you have to supply your pet with enough volume to satisfy the animal's internal stretch receptors (so that it feels full), and at the same time be sure that the volume you're feeding includes all the nutrients your cat needs. One cup of poor-quality food might fill your cat's tummy and supply ample calories, but may not even come close to meeting its nutritional requirements. (See chapter 4 for cat food comparisons.) Keep in mind these numbers are estimates. All cats are unique; while one cat needs 220 calories, another may require only 190.

Mealtime Mistakes

Understanding what they are and how to avoid them

Cats are creatures of habit, and despite the press they've gotten in myth and fable, they are very structure-oriented animals that thrive physically and emotionally on routine, particularly in matters of food and feeding. This type of behavior has its advantages and disadvantages for both owner and pet.

ADVANTAGES	DISADVANTAGES
You decide what, where, when, and how much your cat will eat.	Your cat doesn't always agree with your decisions.
Your cat is secure in knowing where and when it will get its next meal.	Changes in schedule, feeding location, and especially food are not generally greeted with enthusiasm by your cat.
Being smarter than your cat, you can learn to avoid mealtime mistakes, plan ahead for food or schedule changes, and keep your cat in optimal health; making feeding trouble-free for life.	None.

Most Common Feeding Mistakes
Leaving food available at all times*

Cats are no more intrinsic nibblers than humans, and if you have an unlimited quantity of food lying about for either, it's going to be eaten—and eventually in excessive amounts. (See chapter 11 on obesity.)

If you're going to be away for the weekend, leaving dry food for your cat is fine, providing you've also arranged an ample supply of fresh water. Be sure the dry food has at least three meat proteins in the first 6–7 ingredients; that will ensure the urine ph is acidic.

If, because of personal or professional obligations, you must allow your cat to self-feed, provide form and flavor variety right from the start. Cats, if permitted, will easily become addicted to one food, to the exclusion of all others, which can be dangerous and even life threatening, if a dietary change is deemed necessary in the event of an illness.

Do not leave food available for nibbling if you intend to feed one or two balanced meals a day. Except for kittens and pregnant or lactating queens, cats do not need the additional calories of a round-the-clock buffet.

If you have a kitten and know you won't be home in time to serve the next meal until much later, wait until a few minutes after the kitten has eaten his normal meal and then place dry food in his dish. Don't worry if the kitten gobbles this down, too; just refill the bowl. This is not going to be an everyday occurrence, so don't worry. The kitten will probably sleep a lot while you're gone and might not be overly hungry for the next meal, but you'll be assured that he or she will have enough food to eat even if you're delayed in returning.

Canned foods can spoil and cause gastrointestinal ailments if left out all day.

*Only FLUTD-prone cats should have food available at all times unless they are obese.

Feeding only canned food

Though canned meals (see chapter 4) have more protein and fat than dry or moist-packaged foods, you're paying more for palatability and water than for nutrition.

Cats fed only canned or moist-packaged foods are prone to tooth problems (accumulations of tartar), gum inflammation, bad breath, and other periodontal ailments. Some cats love the taste so much they don't chew—they inhale—and soon after, regurgitate.

Over-supplementing with vitamins and minerals

Whether through in natural organ meats or professional vitamin supplements, over-supplementing your pet's diet can cause major health problems. Be particularly careful about vitamins A and D, calcium, and phosphorus. (Check the requirements and overdose cautions in chapter 2.) If you're feeding your cat a quality food, don't add any synthetic supplements that haven't been specifically prescribed. I prefer natural, whole foods or enzymes as a supplement; examples include bee pollen (Dr. Jane® Beezyme), algae, Prozyne, or Florazyme. These won't imbalance the food and counteract its nutritional effectiveness.

Feeding from the same dish

When cats get together, the dominant cat will get the larger portion of food (and nutrients). Even if Godzilla isn't hungry, competitive eating will inspire him to down more than half (if not all) of Peanuts's necessary portion. Keep their dishes separate and in different locations if necessary.

Feeding from plastic dishes

A cat's nose is extremely sensitive, and because plastic is very porous it can retain odors, not all of which might be olfactory turn-ons for your pet. Your cat will turn away from its favorite food if the odor of an unpalatable previous meal is still present. If the plastic has become scraped, bacteria can form in the ridges and cause gastrointestinal problems for your pet. Moreover, some cats are allergic or sensitive to plastic. Symptoms include feline acne or change in nose color.

Hard ceramic or stainless-steel bowls and dishes are easier to keep clean and odor-free. But remember to rinse well! Sometimes even a change in dishwashing soap can cause a keen-nosed cat to spurn a favorite meal; in fact, a really repugnant odor can put a cat off food to the point of starvation. If you want to avoid washing and still maintain cleanliness, paper plates or plastic foam bowls are fine to use, provided they're discarded after each meal and you've secured them (either with a weight or double-stick tape) so your pet won't become frustrated while trying to eat.

CAUTION: Do not wash your cat's feeding dishes with Lysol or strong bleaches. These substances can be toxic to cats, and if any remains on the dish, it could burn your pet's nose or tongue.

Feeding in a noisy or active environment

Many cats are thought to be finicky eaters, or suffering from intestinal distress because of vomiting after eating, when in fact they are only reacting to their feeding location. Usually it's the kitchen and their food is put down for them at the same hectic time the family meal is being prepared.

Cats can lose their appetite with too much noise, too many people, or other pets in their environment.

Feeding raw meat

Yes, cats are carnivores, but just because they'll hunt outdoors and munch on an uncooked field mouse doesn't mean it's desirable for you to serve your pet raw meat. True, some nutrients are destroyed by cooking, but so are many destructive bacteria. Raw meat can contain Toxoplasmosis Ghondii—a parasite that you can get as well as your cat. (Salmonellae can grow quickly on meat and poultry after spending several days in a supermarket cooler before being purchased.) Believe me, it's worth the trade-off, especially where organ meats are concerned, since these are where roundworm larvae are usually found.

I advise cooking all meats until they are at least rare (or to a temperature of 140° to 165° F). For owners who are intent on serving their cats raw meat: there is one complete, balanced raw-meat food that I know is handled properly, it's called Carnivore Connection. There are various formulations available, call 414-248-9256; (1) be sure that meat is promptly refrigerated after it is purchased; (2) rinse the meat with water; (3) feed the meat from the refrigerator—don't leave it at room temperature.

Feeding leftovers

- Table scraps can be added to a cat's regular meal provided they do not make up more than 1/4 of the animal's daily ration.
- Never feed your cat leftovers that you feel are unfit for human consumption.
- Don't feed just one food type.
- Don't feed raw meat, especially poultry or fish.

Giving homemade meals

If the diet is adequately formulated, homemade meals are fine for your pet. Unfortunately, as I've discovered in my treatment of sick cats, adequately formulated homemade meals are a rarity. Before you can say "Din-din is ready," your cat is going to decide what he or she does or doesn't like and become addicted to a particular food to the exclusion of others. That's when feeding and health problems begin.

You have to realize that what's nutritionally good for you is not necessarily adequate for your cat, and vice versa. If we ate the proportional amounts of protein and type of fat that cats need every day, we'd soon be in sad physical shape. On the other hand, there are additives in human foods that are safe for us but can cause major problems for cats.

If you feel you want to give your cat table food, limit the amount. It'll be fun for you and fine for your cat; make it a treat.

Providing too little water

If your cat eats dry food, leaving him a fresh supply of water every day is a necessity. An average seven-pound cat needs 200 ml (milliliters), or about 6–7 ounces, of water daily. The water aids in the metabolism of nutrients for energy, in body temperature maintenance, and in regulating fluid as well as in electrolyte balancing (ionized salts in blood, tissue fluids and cells). With dry food, your pet is getting less than an ounce of water, which is insufficient for just about all of a cat's healthy bodily functions. (See the discussion of water in chapter 2.)

Even though many canned cat foods contain 78 percent water, which would be an ample intake if this were a cat's sole diet (though not one I'd recommend), I'd still advise making fresh or bottled (noncarbonated) water available to your pet. Broth or tomato juice can substitute for fluid intake, but milk cannot. Milk is a food and should not be considered a replacement for fluid. Cats like to play with dripping water—so a slow dripping faucet may help tempt your cat into drinking more water.

Mono-food feeding

Allowing your cat to eat only one food is setting your pet up for a fall from health. Though I've mentioned this before, it bears repeating:

Cats are creatures of habit and can easily become addicted to a particular food to the exclusion of everything else.

Variety, for cats, is not only the spice of life—it's the key to it! No matter what "complete and balanced" food you are feeding your pet, I strongly advise feeding him another brand at least once (preferably two or three times) weekly. Different breeds and different environments, including a variety of stress conditions, create different nutritional needs that no one brand of cat food can cover.

Some brands will have more of certain minerals than others, for instance. By offering your cat minimal variety, you can cover all nutritional bases and provide maximum nutrition. In addition, introducing your pet to various textures and tastes can prevent many problems (and trips to the veterinarian) and often enable simple changes in diet to do the work of expensive medication.

The wrong treats

Bones—chicken bones, fish bones, sparerib bones, any bones that can splinter or break—can become wedged in your pet's mouth or stuck in its throat. Even though your cat may enjoy gnawing on a lamb or beef shank bone, it's still risky. Though the exercise might be great for your pet's gums, a large bone could break some teeth. In any event, after three to four hours without refrigeration, whatever meat is on the bone can develop bacteria, and the bone should be discarded.

Milk is fine for your kittens, but many mature cats are unable to digest it because of a lactose intolerance, and they will develop diar-rhea, which can cause dehydration.

Chocolate, though rich in arginine, an amino acid necessary for cats (see chapter 2) and particularly in the prevention of ammonia in-toxication, is high in the stimulant theobromine. Theobromine can diminish the flow of blood to the brain and kill a cat. A six-ounce bar of chocolate can kill a five-pound cat. If you've allowed your cat to de-velop a liking for chocolate, you would be wise to keep it out of scent range and sealed tightly.

Raw egg white is not good for your cat. Despite all the movies you've seen where athletes add raw eggs to their breakfast drinks, the avidin in raw egg white can deplete your cat of vital biotin (see chapter 2) and undermine your pet's health. Egg yolk (the yellow part) is fine, and so is the white as long as the egg has been cooked. Raw egg can be contaminated with bacteria, so don't serve it to immune-depressed cats.

Holiday cheer, especially in the form of rum-and-brandy-laced eggnog, should never be offered. Your cat might lap a small bit, become tipsy and delight your guests. The amusement will be short-lived, how-ever, if your pet develops a taste for alcohol (which is not uncommon), and takes to seeking it out whenever you have company or a drink. Al-cohol can deplete your cat of all B complex vitamins as well as vitamin C, vitamin K, zinc, magnesium and potassium, to say nothing of caus-ing organ damage, hampering the liver's ability to process fat, and de-stroying brain cells. That's not what I'd call a treat. Avoid spicy food. It often causes diarrhea or vomiting.

Bad timing

Giving your cat commercial kitty treats before meals (to put off having to feed your pet while you relax after coming home from work), or between meals (just as little snacks to show your affec-tion), is a big mealtime mistake. These treats are manufactured to be highly palatable, and your cat will soon be clamoring for more than one—and chances are you'll soon be giving more than one. Not only will this diminish the cat's appetite, causing your pet to eat less of his regular food and, therefore, miss out on nutrients that are re-quired daily, but it can turn tabby tubby if not kept in check.

If you want to show love and affection to your cat, it's not nec-essary to do it with food. Blow bubbles and let your cat jump and break them. Jiggle a string around and watch your cat chase it. Crumple a piece of wrapping paper and let your pet play solo soccer with it. Feeding is a poor substitute for love. Play is a much healthier—and appreciated—alternative.

Giving hair-ball medication before, with, or right after meals is quintessential bad timing. The medicine interferes with vitamin absorption and should be administered between meals! (See chapter 7 for the way to handle and prevent hair balls.)

Owner Precautions for Plant Eaters

If your cat's a plant eater, be sure your plants are safe to eat!

Greens and grasses are sought instinctively by cats for a variety of reasons, but if their selection is limited by environment, cats don't always make the right choices, and protecting them from the wrong plants is up to you.

The Whys and the Wise: Domestic cats usually seek out greens to cleanse their intestines (either of hair balls or foods they wish they hadn't eaten). They do so because of an innate desire for plant matter (which in an undomesticated feline is obtained from the stomach of its prey), a dietary lack of vitamins (particularly vitamin C and the B complex), or—in the case of some house cats—simply out of boredom or to demonstrate their anger at something you've done . . . or haven't done.

Whatever the reason, supplying your cat with safe, nibbleable greens is a wise idea. Eliminating dangerous greens is also wise.

The Goodies

Alfalfa Sprouts

These are a great nutrient source and easy to grow indoors.

Catnip (*Nepeta cataria*)

Some cats enjoy catnip as a zesty, energizing treat; others seem to get happily high on it. They sniff it, lick it, chew it, rub themselves against it and roll around in it. The live plants do not seem to cause the often frenzied behavior that the dried leaves do, and most cats prefer the growing plant to the dried leaves when there is a choice. In fact, they'll usually eat the entire plant. Kittens under three months old tend to ignore catnip, and Siamese cats, as a general rule, are not impressed by it. Then again, it takes a lot to impress a Siamese.

Parsley

This can be grown indoors or in a garden. Fine for cats and for you, too.

Rye or Wheat Grass

This can be planted easily in your garden or obtained from pet stores and grown in an apartment window box. It supplies a lot of antioxidants.

Thyme

Cats enjoy sniffing and nibbling this herb, though it offers none of the stimulant excitement of catnip or valerian. In fact, it often causes quite the opposite reaction, leaving the cat pleasantly laid back and content.

Valerian (*Valeriana officinalis*)

Cats respond to this the way they do to catnip. Interestingly, both valerian and catnip, though outwardly stimulating to cats, are used in internal tranquilizing preparations.

When you grow your own grass, I'd suggest a small pot so that it's too small to act as a litter box. Persians seem to enjoy the coolness of the soil—despite the injury to the growing grass.

The Baddies

Bittersweet

The orange berries are pretty but can be deadly if eaten.

Christmas (Pine) Trees

Keep your pet away from the water stand under the tree. If your cat decides to take a drink, the animal might ingest some pine needles. These contain pine tar, which aside from preventing absorption of vital nutrients, can cause serious gastrointestinal problems.

Dieffenbachia

If you don't know what types of plants are in your home, it's your responsibility as a cat owner to find out. Dieffenbachia, also known as dumb cane and the mother-in-law plant (because if a piece of the stem is put on the tongue or chewed, it can render a person speechless for a short time), has a fast-acting toxicity for cats. It causes labored breathing, severe mouth irritation, and intense abdominal cramps very quickly after ingestion.

Jerusalem Cherry *(Christmas cherry)*

This small bushlike houseplant stays enticingly pretty for weeks with bright red or orange berries, which are highly toxic if ingested and can cause cyanide poisoning.

Laurel *(Sheep Laurel or Mountain Laurel)*

Frequently used in floral arrangements, laurel can poison your pet. If you have any in your home and notice some missing, watch your cat for symptoms such as discharge from eyes and nose, excessive salivation, vomiting, and limb trembling or paralysis. Call your veterinarian quickly if such symptoms are present.

Philodendron and Other Large-Leaf Ivies

These common houseplants are frequently nibbled on by cats, and the effects of repeated ingestion are cumulative. It may take one to three months for symptoms of poisoning (see above) to appear.

Poinsettias

Although poinsettias are holiday beauties in any home, they are dangerous for greens-seeking cats. The leaves can cause skin, eye, mouth, and stomach inflammations.

Other Leaves Your Cat Should Leave Alone:

Arrowgrass	Locoweed
Azalea	Mistletoe
Hemlock	Oleander
Jimsonweed	Peach Leaves
Larkspur	Rhubarb Leaves
Lily of the Valley	Wisteria

New-Life Preventive Nutrition Tactics

A fortified immune system can help your cat fight back.

When a cat's diet is imbalanced or inadequate, so is the animal's immune system—the defense force necessary for warding off illness, protecting against toxins, healing injuries, mobilizing energy, and preserving good health. Since you're in charge of your pet's diet, the strength of that defense force depends on you!

Preventive Ammunition: Today's cats are exposed to more toxic substances than ever before, which is why they need more high-powered immune-building nutrients in their diets.

Adding extra vitamin C and E to your cat's daily fare is a simple and smart dietary safeguard. (See chapter 2 for best sources and ways to administer.)

If your cat is in good health and eats a high-quality food regularly, (see chapter 4), or is currently on my New-Life Diet (see chapter 10), an additional supplement of 100 mg of vitamin C, 50 mg of vitamin B complex, and 30 IU of vitamin E daily is an optional, but advisable, immune-system booster.

Our cats may have two disadvantages that we need to overcome.

1. The lack of adequate antioxidants in their diet. Pet food manufacturers have not embraced the importance of antioxidants yet; in fact they still believe that cats produce enough vitamin C so that additional amounts in the food are not required.

2. The lack of "natural," non-altered nutrients in their diet that their ancestors got from nibbling on different plants and eating small animals. Our cat foods are formulated based on the common ingredients used for more than 50 years in the pet food industry: corn, soy, meat, dairy, etc. While these ingredients provide our cats with substantial nutrition, they are void of many of the food components found in plants and whole animals. Scientists are currently studying many of these various micronutrients, demonstrating their tremendous medicinal and preventive properties. Aloe vera, which I recommend for constipation, has more than 200 components that all work together to produce the wondrous effects of the plant. Many of these micronutrient components, as with other herbs, are simply not present in cat food or cat treats—and the only way our cats can get them is through supplementation.

What and How to Supplement for a Fortified Immune System

Since there is no question that you should be adding a supplement to your cat's daily fare, you must determine which one is best. The type and frequency of supplementation will depend on you and your cat.

Daily Vitamin, Mineral Supplement

If you are feeding a brand-name supermarket food, I suggest you add a daily vitamin/mineral supplement that will help ensure a full supply of nutrients, including amino acids and fatty acids. The following are brands I recommend:

1. Pro Balance   Amino acids, fatty acids, vitamins and minerals—sold by veterinarians only.
2. F Biotic   Wysong—Amino acids, fatty acids, probiotic, herbs, vitamins, and minerals.
3. Nu-cat   Vitamins, minerals, enzymes, fatty acids, and sea mussels. Sold by veterinarians only (Vetri science: 1-800-882-9993).

4. Dr. Jane® Beezyme   Bee pollen plus vegetable enzymes (1-800-DR
                       JANE B).

If you are feeding a professional alternative-brand cat food, then your
supplement should be a complete food (herb) or an enzyme supplement.
A prepared vitamin/mineral supplement has the potential to upset the
balance of the manufactured cat food, while a complete food or vegetable
enzyme (Prozyme or Florazyme) will not. In fact, many of these foods will
state that supplementation is not advised. Supplements I recommend for
a professional alternative food include:

1. Dr. Jane® Beezyme   Bee pollen plus vegetable enzymes.
OR
2. Bee pollen
AND/OR
3. Prozyme   Vegetable enzymes studied at the Mayo
                        Clinic Laboratories (1-800-522-5537).

AND/OR
4. Florazyme   Vegetable enzyme and probiotics
                        (305-739-4416).

AND/OR
5. Algae

Antioxidants

These should be added to your cat's fare even if you are using a daily
vitamin/mineral supplement. The choice of antioxidants is yours. You can
use vitamin C and E (they are more effective when used together), or antioxidant formulations (containing multiple antioxidants).

1. Dr. Jane® Feline Formula One (1-800-Dr Jane B)
OR
2. Super C Complex
   (Nutra Pet) (1-800-221-0308)
AND/OR
3. Herbs—which include wheat grass, parsley or algae.
AND/OR
4. Ester C (1-800-274-7387)

AND/OR
5. Prime of Life Antioxidant (manufactured for Fit n' Frisky Products Inc., Cheyenne, WY 82001)

Other Supplements

Supplements that I recommend for dull coats, dry skin and skin lesions include fatty acids and B vitamins:
1. Dr. Jane® Essential Gold (1-800-Dr Jane B)
2. Opticoat II (1-800-548-2899)
3. Derm Caps (sold by veterinarians only)
4. Brewer's or torula yeast and/or a multi-B complex vitamin
5. Dr. Jane® Feline Formula One

Amounts of Supplement

ADULT CATS
VITAMIN B COMPLEX
50–75 mg daily
OR
1/4 teaspoon torula or brewer's yeast
VITAMIN C
50–100 mg Ester C daily
VITAMIN E
30 IU daily (or 1/4 teaspoonful wheat germ)

HERBAL ENZYMATIC SUPPLEMENT
1/4 teaspoon Dr. Jane® Beezyme or bee pollen daily in food
AND/OR
1/4 to 1/8 teaspoon Prozyme or Florazyme
AND/OR
Home-grown wheat grass in a flower pot for daily nibbling

AGING CATS (over 6 years)
VITAMIN B COMPLEX
50–75 mg daily
OR
1/4 teaspoon torula or brewer's yeast (can mix bran into this)

VITAMIN C
100–150 mg Ester C daily (Natural Animal 1-800-274-7387)

VITAMIN E
15–30 IU units daily (can be divided in two doses daily with meals)

HERBAL ENZYMATIC SUPPLEMENT
1/4 teaspoonful Dr. Jane® Beezyme or bee pollen twice daily in food
1/4 to 1/8 teaspoon Prozyme or Florazyme daily
1/4 teaspoon wheat grass infusion daily
Wheat grass in a flower pot for nibbling
1/8 to 1/4 teaspoon algae daily

PREGNANT OR LACTATING CATS

For pregnant cats only
1/4 dropper red raspberry infusion or tea daily. Should be started at
40th to 50th day.

For both pregnant and/or lactating cats
VITAMIN B COMPLEX
75–100 mg daily
OR
TORULA OR BREWER'S YEAST
1/4 teaspoon

VITAMIN E
30 mg daily (can be divided)

HERBAL ENZYMATIC SUPPLEMENT
1/4 teaspoon Beezyme® or bee pollen twice daily in food
1/4 to 1/8 teaspoon Prozyme or Florazyme
Wheat grass in a flower pot for nibbling

FOR KITTENS OVER 3 MONTHS OLD

VITAMIN B COMPLEX
50 mg daily

BREWER'S YEAST
1/8 teaspoon

HERBAL ENZYMATIC SUPPLEMENT
1/8 teaspoon Dr. Jane® Beezyme or bee pollen daily in food
1/8 teaspoon Prozyme or Florazyme

Wheat grass in a flower pot for nibbling

Note that I do not include vitamin C. It may interfere with complete bone growth and is, therefore, only recommended for sick kittens.

Q&A

Feline Urinary Tract Health

My two male cats have had reoccurring problems with FUS (Feline Urologic Syndrome). I understand that it is now called FLUTD (Feline Lower Urinary Tract Disease), and that it can kill a cat within 1–2 days. It seems that for some reason, crystals or plugs build up in the urine of the cat, creating a blockage, which does not allow the cat to urinate. I'd like to know what causes this disease, and if females can get it as well as males? Is it the same thing as cystitis?

This complex disease, which probably has many causes, including allergy, stress, breed, overweight and perhaps even virus, is found in both male and female cats. Because of the male anatomy, owners tend to notice urination problems in males easier than in females (bloody urine, straining to urinate). Cystitis is an inflammation of the bladder, and yes, it can be part of the complex disease. We suspect that foods producing alkaline urines (basic, rather than acidic), help magnesium accumulate in the urinary tract. We currently recommend foods that produce an acidic urine (pH of 6.1–6.4) with a magnesium content of no more than .1 percent on a dry matter basis or no more than .02 percent in canned food.

When supplementing your cat's diet, you must keep in mind magnesium content. Brewer's yeast has a higher magnesium level than torula yeast, yet they are rather similar in taste and nutritional properties.

Meat produces an acidic urine while cereal produces the opposite. When buying cat food, look for meat proteins. Some veterinarians recommend tomato sauce or adding vitamin C to keep the urine acidic, while others don't feel that it works. My feeling is to give it a try; it can't hurt if you don't give too much.

Calorie Confusion

I'm a new (and conscientious) cat owner, but I just don't understand the difference between calories, kilocalories, and k-cals. I'd like to be sure my cat is getting his proper daily caloric intake, but I don't know how many calories are in a k-cal. Is there a simple conversion formula?

Very simple. None. For your purposes (and the purpose of this book), a calorie is a kilocalorie and a k-cal. Whether your cat needs 40 calories, kilocalories, or k-cals per pound of body weight daily, if he weighs eight pounds, he's going to need 240 of any one (or all) of them.

What's important to remember is that the calories in a cup of dry food and a cup of can food—or a cup of leftovers—are not the same.

Sloppy Eater

I always thought cats were neat and clean, but my two-year-old mixed breed tiger-striped cat, Sheena, can't eat a meal without splattering food on the wall or floor. Oh, she'll lick herself clean afterward, but I'm left with washing the baseboard and mopping up the floor. Is she being hostile, or what? And is there anything I can do about it?

You could start by putting her food in a deeper feeding dish, and then placing that dish away from the wall on newspaper, or switch her to a dry food. I doubt she's being hostile. It sounds as if she's really hungry and gobbling her food quickly. Maybe if you fed her earlier—or more often—she would slow down.

Living with a Leaf Lover

My cat snacks on my house plant leaves as if they were after-dinner mints. I give her a pet vitamin daily, so I can't believe she has a nutritional deficiency. She also gets lots of love and attention. Have you any idea why she does this? And any suggestions for saving my plants?

I can think of numerous reasons why your cat might be a leaf nibbler, but you will have to zero in on the right one. She might need
more non-digestible fiber in her diet (such as beet pulp, oat bran or
Psillium) to cleanse her intestines. Combine equal amounts of oat
bran, brewer's or torula yeast and sprinkle less than 1/8 teaspoon on
her food, increasing daily to 1/4 teaspoon. Try giving her a salad once
in a while and see what happens.

On the other hand, her attraction for your plants might be nothing more than the motion of the leaves (from a breeze, fan or whatever), which excites her hunting instinct.

As for saving your plants, you can buy cat repellent sprays at pet
stores that might help. Other than that, all I can suggest is to hang
your plants from the ceiling and hope for the best.

No Can Do

Is it all right for me to feed my cat food directly from the can?

I don't recommend it. There's no harmful substance in the can
(such as lead), but after you open it with a can opener there might be
jagged edges around the top that could injure your pet's mouth or
tongue. And because the can is light, your cat will have difficulty eating, most likely spending its mealtime pushing and chasing its dinner
around the room.

Dishing It Out

*I was told that I shouldn't leave my cat's water bowl right next to his food
dish. Why not?*

Because cats use their tongues to get food into their mouths, and
don't always do so neatly, so food remnants can easily drop into the
water, spoil, and contaminate it. That is the reason I'm not in favor of
those double feeding dishes with one side for water and the other for
food. A little distance between the food and water dishes is all that's
necessary, and don't forget to keep the water fresh.

Part Two

....

Feeding the Right Stuff

....

CHAPTER 4

······················

Let's Talk
Cat Food

······················

Cat Food Categories Simplified

What makes the difference

In the vast kingdom of pet foods there are two basic categories: supermarket/commercial food and alternative food. Since they are often misunderstood, and I refer to them frequently throughout the book, it's important that you understand their differences.

Supermarket/Commercial Food

The pet food industry is valued at about five billion dollars, with everyone trying to get in on the profit. Major-brand supermarket foods have been part of this industry for over forty years, creating tasty, affordable food that will deliver adequate, balanced nutrition. Since these companies compete by advertising extensively on television and in magazines, cost is often reduced via the ingredients in the food.

Ingredients may vary in quality and amount depending on the ups and downs of the commodities market—categorizing these foods as "non-fixed ingredient foods." You may buy a particular brand of chicken dinner today, and find that the same food next week has a little more cereal and a different type of chicken. This may not bother all cats, but stressed, sick, reproducing or sensitive cats can have a difficult time with these modifications in the formulas.

Cat food ingredients are expensive, especially meats (chicken, fish, beef, poultry by-products, etc.) and good quality fats. In order to reduce the cost of the food, many of these manufacturers use cereal proteins such as soy, corn gluten, rice gluten, wheat or barley rather than meats. While these cereals can be formulated to give adequate nutrition that is usually tested to be balanced, the types of proteins and fats used rarely result in the types of health that breeders and veterinarians expect. You must understand that there is NOTHING WRONG with the major-brand supermarket foods; it's just that they have different standards for healthy cats. Dandruff, dry or oily skin, matted coats, and large stools are acceptable. Most foods pass the AAFCO (American Association of Feed Control Officials) food testing, which requires the manufacturer to feed the food to cats, with the cats passing a physical exam and basic blood work indicating a normal cat. The condition of muscles, skin, coat, immune system, etc., simply are not major factors. Supermarket-brand cat food can be analogous to Burger King: it's tasty and delivers nutrition, but it's just not the same type of nutrition you get from a premium piece of meat with fresh vegetables.

Alternative Food

Shiny, long, full coats with small non-odorous stools are generally a result of higher quality meat proteins and fats. Food companies that are willing to invest in this higher level of nutrition need to sell their products for more, and thus place them in places where ingredients can be explained to the consumer: pet shops, feed stores, health food shops, breeders and veterinarian offices.

There are many food companies that have entered this market, some of them using better ingredients than others and some of them actually studying feline nutrition (a relatively new science), employing nutritionists and veterinarians, funding studies in universities, and funding testing of nutrient levels from blood, fecal and urine tests in cats that are fed these foods.

Professional Alternative Food Companies

Professional alternative food companies are those manufacturers that have "fixed ingredients," and do ongoing studies, besides the AAFCO feeding tests to be certain the nutrients they use are, in fact, of high quality and available to the cat.

Non-Professional Alternative Food Companies

Non-professional alternative foods are also sold in these same alternative markets. They generally use meat ingredients rather than cereal and higher levels of fat. Results of feeding these foods include shiny coats, healthier-looking bodies and smaller stools. These foods are priced similar to professional companies. Alternative food companies may or may not make their own food (the label will say "manufactured for"), and they certainly don't spend money on testing and researching ingredients and food. (I would rather have my cat's food thoroughly tested.) Most of them do comply with what I consider to be the minimum requirements: they perform the AAFCO feeding tests, feeding the food to cats, and determining specific parameters.

Needless to say, I would rather have you feed a professional alternative food rather than a non-professional food. Labels, bags, and cans won't tell you if you are feeding a professional or non-professional food. You have to call the manufacturer and ask about their studies, how many nutritionists and veterinarians are on staff and with which universities are they working. I consider Hills, Iams, Proplan and Waltham professional alternative companies.

The Four Cat Food Types Explained

Know your options for optimal cat health.

There are four types of food for cats: canned, semi-moist, dry and homemade. (I'm excluding such occasional feline fast foods as birds, mice, moles and so on, since I consider these random and circumstantial choices that only cats—and not their owners—make.)

Understanding what these foods are, their nutritional and economic advantages and disadvantages, and deciding what they offer your cat in the way of health as well as what they offer you in the way of convenience are essential for the successful revitalization and lifetime fitness of your pet.

Canned Food

Advantages
- High in fat; more palatable than dry food.
- Contains more digestible meat proteins than most dry food.
- Has a high caloric density, which means your cat can easily meet daily energy requirements.
- Food is cooked in the can, destroying potential disease-causing bacteria.
- Has a longer shelf life than dry or semi-moist food.
- Has less chance of insect or bacterial infestation than other types of food.
- Doesn't necessarily need preservatives.

Disadvantages
- High moisture content, which means you're paying a lot of money for water. For cats with FLUTD this is an advantage, since increased liquid intake is recommended.
- Food-processing heat causes loss of nutrients.
- Many brands contain color additives (for aesthetic appeal to owners), some of which could be carcinogenic (cancer-causing). All have the potential to adversely affect a cat's physical and emotional health.
- Many manufacturers disguise TVP (textured vegetable protein) so that it looks like animal protein.
- Needs refrigeration after opening.

Semi-moist Food

Advantages
- Comes in convenient, easy-to-serve pouches or cans.
- Doesn't spoil if left out, the way canned food does.
- Because of processing techniques, semi-moist food can contain

more added nutrients than canned food, but not as many as dry food.

- Quite palatable, but not as palatable as canned food.
- Has a higher caloric density than canned or dry food because of its sugar and/or carbohydrate content. These are used to prevent bacteria and fungi formation, as well as to retain moisture. This is useful in the control of diarrhea.

Disadvantages

- Contains a variety of artificial colorings, some of which could be carcinogenic (cancer-causing), and all of which could adversely affect a cat's physical and emotional well-being.
- Costs more than equivalent cat foods.
- High in salt and magnesium.
- Difficult to switch cats off of this and onto healthier foods.

Dry Food

Advantages

- Low in moisture with a high concentration of nutrients.
- Cheaper than canned food.
- Doesn't require refrigeration; easily stored.
- Can be left in the cat's feeding dish all day without spoiling.
- Can promote dental health by decreasing tartar accumulation.
- Generally has a better nutritional analysis than canned food, because of the lower water content.
- Great way to feed pregnant cats or kittens.

Disadvantages

- Highly vulnerable to pathogens (microorganisms or substances, such as molds, insects and fungi, which are capable of causing disease).
- Supermarket brands are frequently lower in fat and, therefore, less palatable than canned food.
- Supermarket brands are frequently higher in cereal content and difficult for many cats to digest.
- Any nutrient to which a cat could react adversely may be ten times more concentrated in dry form. On the other hand, any nutrient to which a cat responds favorably could be ten times more effective.

- With the exception of some alternative brands, mineral content is often too high, particularly in salt and magnesium.
- Owners tend to leave food out all day for free feeding, which can create a finicky eater and cause obesity. I am totally against free feeding unless you have a kitten in need of food when you can't be there, have a sick cat, have a cat prone to FLUTD or are going away and have no one to feed your pet.
- Some of the cereal-based dry foods have added acid to artificially promote acidic urines, which can create possible medical problems for your cat.

Homemade Food

These are meals made from an owner's recipes with the owner's selection of ingredients.

Advantages
- Ingredients are readily available and protein is usually of higher biological value quality with fewer artificial-flavor additives.
- Recipes can be tailored to a cat's individual needs.
- Generally very palatable.

Disadvantages
- Recipes are frequently imbalanced and deficient in necessary nutrients.

Table Scraps

These are meals made solely from the leftovers of family meals, usually all meat.

Advantages
- Inexpensive and convenient.

Disadvantages
- Meals are imbalanced, deficient in adequate nutrients, frequently all meat and generally detrimental to a cat's health.

What to Look for on a Cat Food Label

Getting the most for your cat and your money

1. A National Brand Manufacturer

The label should say "manufactured by . . . ," and give the manufacturer's address. If the label says "distributed by . . . ," or "manufactured for . . . ," the food can be of inferior nutritional quality and the formulations are probably not fed and tested except for minimum requirements. (Unfortunately, low-priced food generally means low-quality nutrition.) For your cat's sake, check it out. Write to the manufacturer and ask the following questions:

What is the protein utilization of your food?

Even though the ingredients might be there, you want to know if the food was processed correctly, whether ample vitamins and minerals were included for adequate utilization of those ingredients, and whether the named nutrient percentages are what your pet is actually getting. Think of it this way: even a meat loaf with prime ingredients can be cooked to nutritional destruction. Ask if the manufacturer feeds the food and measures urine and feces (what goes in should not go out).

What is the total protein digestibility of your food?

You want to know if the protein sources (which might be identical to those listed in other brands) are of better quality and, therefore, offer a higher digestibility.

What is the caloric density of your food?

You should know how many calories there are in a can, a cup, or a pound, so that you can adjust your pet's meals accordingly.

What is the urine pH after eating the food?
See information about FLUTD.

Ask for the names of the veterinarians and nutritionists on staff.
The more the better.

Do they fund university studies? Which ones?

Do they have colonies of cats to test liver, kidney, taurine, bones, etc.? Where is the product tested?
     You want to know that all the ingredients have been tested for purity and quality—before and after processing—and that they have the facilities to do such testing. The more extensively they study their food's effect on the cat, the better their food is apt to be.

2. Nutritional Guarantee
     The label should state that the food has undergone AAFCO (American Association of Feed Control Officials) feeding trials and is complete and balanced for all life stages or for adults only.

3. Guaranteed Analysis
     The percentages of nutrients in the food are usually listed above, below, or next to the ingredients on cat food labels. Protein and fat are usually given in minimum amounts since they are the most expensive ingredients. But a large minimum guarantee of protein does not mean that the product's protein is going to be of high biological value quality. Algae, corn gluten, cottonseed, wheat, soybean meals, and others are classified as "plant proteins," which can boost the protein percentages on labels without providing equivalent nutrient benefits—especially for cats, who require animal protein.
     A close ratio of fat to protein is your best indicator of the usable protein your pet is getting. For example, a dry food with a crude protein minimum of 30 percent and a crude fat minimum of 20 percent is a better choice than one with a crude protein minimum of 30 percent and a crude fat minimum of 10 percent.
     Keep in mind that without a substantial amount of fat, the food's calorie content will be so low that excessive amounts will have to be eaten just to meet the cat's daily energy requirements.

Quick Guide to Health Buys

Dry Food

- Minimum protein should be 30 to 35 percent.
- Minimum fat should be at least 15 percent.
- Maximum ash should be no more than 8 percent.*
- Maximum moisture should not be more than 10 percent.

*A "low ash" content does not mean that the food is necessarily low in magnesium, which could be a contributing factor in FLUTD. Magnesium content should not exceed 0.10 percent.

Canned Food

- Minimum protein should be 10 to 12 percent.
- Minimum fat should be at least 3 percent.
- Maximum ash should be no more than 4 percent.*
- Maximum moisture should not be more than 78 percent (simply because you'll be paying more for water than nutrition).

*A "low ash" content does not mean that the food is necessarily low in magnesium, which could be a contributing factor in FLUTD. Magnesium content should not exceed 0.02 percent.

Soft-Moist Food

- Minimum protein should be 24 percent.
- Minimum fat should be 8.5 percent.
- Maximum moisture should not be more than 34 percent.
- Ash content should not exceed 7 percent.

4. Ingredients

Each ingredient in a pet food must be listed on the product label in descending order by weight to provide a general indication of the product's content and quality.

The first four ingredients listed should contain at least two sources of high biological value protein (such as meat, fish, poultry or cheese).

In the entire ingredient panel, there should be:
- no more than three digestible carbohydrates.
- some source of animal fat (if not specifically listed and the protein/fat ratio is close, a sufficient amount is usually present).
- a long list of vitamins and minerals (the longer the better).
- no artificial coloring.

(See "Understanding Ingredients" below.)

And my personal advice is to avoid any cat foods containing:

Gluten meal

The protein part of processed wheat, corn, and other carbohydrates, gluten meal can cause a malabsorption of food from the intestinal tract (gluten enteropathy) and a variety of intestinal problems.

Whey

This is the liquid left after the curd and cream are separated from milk. It can cause intestinal problems in cats with a lactose intolerance.

Peanut hulls

Hulls are the outer covering of peanuts. They are a poor form of fiber, offer zero nutrition and can cause many feline intestinal problems.

Wheat shorts

This is the residue of wheat processing and milling. It represents a poor supply of fiber that can cause intestinal problems as well as nutritional deficiencies.

Dyes

Dyes can cause sensitivity (diarrhea, feline acne).

Understanding Ingredients

You don't have to pronounce them, but you should know what they are if your cat is eating them.

Because of man-made feed components and labeling technicalities, looking at cat food ingredients and trying to figure out which are proteins and which are carbohydrates, which are vitamins and which are additives, is not easy. Since this knowledge is essential to evaluating a food as well as to increasing your pet's health, the following category breakdown of ingredients should simplify things.

Most Common Cat Food Ingredients

High Biological Value Protein Sources

Meat (flesh from beef, pork, goat, lamb, mutton; may include skeletal muscle, flesh from tongue, esophagus, diaphragm and heart)

Beef	Whole egg
Liver	Poultry giblets
Kidney	Poultry by-products
Ocean whitefish	Liver meal
Tuna	Chicken
Beef by-products	Meat by-products
Fish meal	Meat meal
Poultry by-products meal	Glandular meal

Backup Protein Sources to Boost Protein Content

Fish solubles	Textured vegtable protein
Hydrolyzed poultry feathers	(TVP)
Digest (liquefied, chemically	Soy flour
predigested meat)	Whey
Soybean meal	

Amino Acids (Essential Components of Protein)

L-Lysine	MHA
DL-Methionine	

Fat Sources

Chicken fat	Soybean oil
Wheat germ oil	Cod-liver oil
Animal fat	Safflower oil
Fish oil	Flax seed oil

Carbohydrates (Digestible)

Brewer's rice
Rice flour
Corn gluten meal
Cornmeal
Flax meal

Ground yellow corn
Wheat flour
Wheat germ meal
Ground corn
Barley

Carbohydrates (Non-Digestible)

Beet pulp
Tomato pomace
Rice hulls

Cellulose
Peanut hulls

Preservatives and Additives

Sodium nitrite..........(preservative and color fixative; may be carcinogenic)

Sodium nitrate.........(may be carcinogenic)

MSG......................(monosodium glutamate; a concentrated source of sodium)

BHA ....(butylated hydroxyanisole; a chemical preservative to keep food from becoming rancid)

BHT ....(butylated hydroxytoluene; excess can adversely affect kidneys)

Ethoxyquin ....(chemical preservative)

Caramel coloring .....(artificial coloring; an additive)

Guar gum.................(a binder; plant carbohydrate)

Vegetable gums........(binders; plant carbohydrates)

Benzoic acid.............(chemical preservative)

Propyl gallate ....(chemical preservative; may be a cause of liver damage)

Citric acid.................(chemical preservative)

Ascorbic acid............(preservative; also vitamin C)

Titanium dioxide .....(a food coloring)

Vitamins

Brewer's yeast ....(excellent source of multiple
B vitamins)
Pyridoxine/Pyridoxine
hydrochloride.......................(vitamin B_6)
Vitamin A acetate/Vitamin A
palmitate ....(vitamin A)
Choline/Choline chloride...(member of the B complex)
Inositol...............................(member of the B complex)
a-Tocopherol/DL-alpha ....(source of vitamin E)
Tocopherol acetate..............(source of vitamin E; an antioxidant)
Thiamine/Thiamine
mononitrate........................(vitamin B_1)
Riboflavin...........................(vitamin B_2)
Ascorbic acid.......................(vitamin C; also classified as
a preservative)
Folic acid............................(member of the B complex)
Niacin/Niacinamide/
Nicotinamide ....(vitamin B_3)
D-activated animal sterol....(source of vitamin D_3)
Biotin ....(member of B complex)
Menadione/Menadione
sodium bisulfite complex ...(source of vitamin K)
Cyanocobalamin
concentrate ....(source of vitamin B_{12})
Calcium D-pantothenate/
d-Calcium pantothenate.....(vitamin B_{15})
Para-aminobenzoic acid......(member of the B complex)
Lecithin..............................(needed in fat digestion)

Mineral Sources

Calcium carbonate/
Calcium iodate ....(calcium)
Sodium/Sodium
tripolyphosphate.................(salt)

Ferrous sulfate.....................(iron)
Potassium chloride..............(potassium)
Manganese sulfate...............(manganese)
Manganous oxide................(manganese)
Zinc oxide ....(zinc)
Iron carbonate/Iron sulfate (iron)
Copper oxide ....(copper)
Cobalt carbonate.................(cobalt)
Ethylene diamine
dihydroiodide ....(iodine)
EDDI...................................(iodine)
Bonemeal ....(phosphorus and calcium)
Sodium selenite...................(selenium)
Phosphoric acid ....(phosphorus with fluorine)
Defluorinated phosphate......(phosphorus with low fluorine)
Sorbic acid ....(chemical preservative)
Potassium sorbate ....(chemical preservative)

How to Examine Cat Food for Quality

The Home Test for Dry Food

- Fill a glass with water and drop a piece of dry food into it. As it dissolves, watch what comes out. You don't want to see a lot of chicken feathers or hair.
- Check for consistency of size, shape, and density of pellets. They should be uniform. Each piece contains a certain amount of nutrients, and if some of the pieces crush to powder between your fingers while others remain rock hard or vary in size, the manufacturer's extruding equipment (which makes the pellets) is poor, and the product is not likely to be any better.
- Beware of dry food bags that feel greasy on the outside. If the fat has soaked through, the food has been left susceptible to rodent, insect and bacteria infestation.
- See if the food contains a large amount of "fines" (tiny crumb-like particles). A little in any dry food is to be expected; a lot means that the food is not of high quality.

- Smell the food. It should not have a peculiar, moldy or rancid odor.
- Examine the food for color consistency. Any greenish, bluish, blackish or pale pellets in an otherwise color-consistent batch could indicate mold.
- Check the bag's contents for any foreign material, such as rodent waste, paper and insects. Be particularly careful about insects. Many owners feel it's just another source of protein; but some insects have tiny porcupinelike barbs that can damage a cat's esophagus. Take my advice and don't bother to put the insect under a microscope—get the bag of food out of your house.
- Natural, dry food has a shelf life of nine months. Artificially preserved food can last one year. Once opened, it should be stored in a sealed container and kept no longer than two months.

The Home Test for Canned Food

- Be sure that there is no swelling or raised bump on the can. Both usually indicate that the vacuum processing has been broken, and the product can be harboring disease-causing bacteria.
- For a large can, open both ends and push the food onto a platter (or use three small plates). Cut the food into thirds (top, middle, bottom) and compare the three sections. All three sections should have a homogeneous consistency: equal distributions of fat and other ingredients should be evident.
- For small cans, or those with stewlike consistency, put the food on a plate and examine it. You don't want to see large pieces of blood vessels, tendons or ligaments. (These are not high-BV protein meat by-products.) You also don't want to see a large glob of fat in the middle. Fat should be well-distributed throughout. In small cans, fat sometimes rises to the top; this is all right. It's the big glob of poor-quality fat that you want to avoid. There should be no hair, feathers, or any other foreign material in the food.
- Refrigerate the unused portion of canned food, but do not keep it longer than two days.
- Shelf life is generally two years—unopened.

The Home Test for Soft-Moist Food

- Be sure that the package is tightly sealed. Any small tear makes contents an easy target for contamination.
- Soft-moist pellets should be uniformly soft. When crumbled between your fingers, you should not feel crunchy hulls or crackly, fibrous substances.

How Do Name Brands Stack Up?

To help you in selecting the cat foods you want to feed, I have compiled a comprehensive list of major brand cat food manufacturers, supermarket and alternative. I have gathered the data to help you evaluate foods according to the information presented in this chapter. Food companies often change ingredients and/or the usage of them, so while we strive to be exact, the information presented may be out-dated. Toll-free numbers are supplied so you can contact the manufacturer to ask for additional information besides gross analysis, major ingredients, calories and pH.

Remember that the development of a food may start with ingredients and percentages, but the quality of the food also depends on many other variables that a wise owner will check out before feeding that food. I did not include the words maximum or minimum in the gross analysis. Some of the values are listed "as fed," while others are listed "dry matter."

HILLS SCIENCE DIET®
Hills Pet Products
Colgate Palmolive
P.O. Box 148
Topeka, Kansas 66601
1-800-445-5777

Formulations: (canned, dry) Science Diet® Feline Maintenance, Science Diet® Feline Growth, Science Diet® Feline Maintenance Light, Science Diet® Feline Senior, Prescription Diets (through veterinarian's prescription only)

Science Diet® Feline Maintenance® (dry)—AAFCO-tested for adults
   Varieties: Original, Beef, Turkey, Sea Food

Science Diet® Feline Maintenance® (dry) original
   Ingredients: poultry by-products meal, ground corn, brewer's
   rice, animal fat (preserved with BHA, propyl gallate, citric
   acid), corn gluten meal, chicken liver digest

   Protein 30.90%   **Fat** 21.10%   **Fiber** .90%   **Ash** 5.10%
   Magnesium .07%   **Moisture** 7.6%   **Calories** 534 per cup
   Urine pH 6.1–6.4   **Feeding:** 10-pound cat, 1/2 cup daily; or
   1/4 cup dry, 1/4 can

Science Diet® Feline Growth® (dry)—AAFCO-tested for growth
   Ingredients: poultry by-products meal, ground corn, animal fat
   (preserved with BHA, propyl gallate, citric acid), corn gluten
   meal, dried whole egg, chicken liver digest, soy bean mill run

   Protein 33.90%   **Fat** 24.60%   **Fiber** 1.10%   **Ash** 6.0%
   Magnesium .03%   **Moisture** 7.50%   **Calories** 555 per cup
   Urine pH 6.1–6.4   **Feeding:** free feed

Science Diet® Light Formula Feline Maintenance®(dry)—AAFCO-tested for adults
   Ingredients: brewer's rice, poultry by-products meal, corn
   gluten meal, powdered cellulose, animal fat (preserved with
   BHA, propyl gallate, citric acid), chicken liver digest

   Protein 36.90%   **Fat** 8.30%   **Fiber** 6.30%   **Ash** 5.30%
   Magnesium .06%   **Moisture** 9%   **Calories** 243 Kcal per cup
   Urine pH 6.1–6.4   **Feeding:** 10-pound cat, 7/8 cup daily

Science Diet® Light Formula Feline Maintenance® (canned), original—AAFCO-tested for adults
   Ingredients: water, meat by-products, liver, chicken, rice flour,
   glandular meal, brewer's rice, powdered cellulose

   Protein 11.0%   **Fat** 6.2%   **Fiber** .06–.07%   **Ash** 1.5- 1.6%
   Magnesium 0.01–0.02%   **Moisture** 75.5–75.9%
   Calories 171 Kcal per 5 1/2 oz. can   **Urine pH** 6.1–6.4
   Feeding: average cat, one 5 1/2 oz. can daily

Science Diet® Feline Maintenance® (canned), seafood—AAFCO-tested for adults

Ingredients: water, fish, meat by-products, liver, beef, ground corn, animal fat, powdered cellulose

Protein 11.0%   **Fat** 6.2%   **Fiber** 0.6–0.7%   **Ash** 1.5–1.6%
Magnesium 0.01%–0.02%   **Moisture** 75.5–75.9%
Calories 170 Kcal per 5 1/2 oz. can   **Urine pH** 6.1–6.2

Science Diet® Feline Growth® (canned)—AAFCO-tested for growth

Ingredients: water, liver, chicken, egg product, poultry by-products meal, soybean meal, rice, ground corn

Protein 14.80%   **Fat** 10.90%   **Fiber** .20%   **Ash** 2.10%
Moisture 69.3%   **Magnesium** .03%
Calories 258 Kcal per 5 1/2 oz. can
Feeding: kittens, one pound: feed 3/8 of 5 1/2 oz. can; kittens, three pounds: feed 7/8 of 5 1/2 oz. can

Science Diet® Feline Light® (canned)—AAFCO-tested for adults

Ingredients: meat by-products, water, liver, ground corn, powdered cellulose, corn gluten meal

Protein 11.40%   **Fat** 4.40%   **Fiber** 1.60%   **Ash** 1.50%
Magnesium 0.01%   **Moisture** 75%
Calories 164 Kcal per 5 1/2 oz. can   **Urine pH** 6.1–6.4
Feeding: 3/8 of 5 1/2 oz. can

Science Diet® Feline Senior® (canned)—AAFCO-tested for adults

Varieties: Beef formula, Turkey formula

Science Diet Feline Senior® (canned) Beef Formula

Ingredients: water, beef, liver, ground corn, animal fat, glandular meal, powdered cellulose, guar gum, xantham gum, locust bean gum

Protein 10.1–10.2%   **Fat** 5.10%   **Fiber** 1.30%   **Ash** 1.30%
Magnesium 0.1-0.2%   **Moisture** 75.1%
Calories 162 Kcal per 5 1/2 oz. can
Feeding: 10-pound cat, 1 1/2 cans (5 1/2 oz.)

Prescription Diet® Feline c/d® (dry)

Ingredients: brewer's rice, poultry by-product meal, animal fat (preserved with BHA, propyl gallate and citric acid), corn gluten meal, dried whole egg, chicken liver digest

Protein 32%   **Fat** 23.50%   **Fiber** 1.60%   **Magnesium** .054%
Calories 548 per cup   **Moisture** 1.47%   **Urine pH** 6.2–6.4
Feeding: as per your veterinarian's directions

Prescription Diet® Feline c/d® (canned)
Ingredients: meat by-products, water, liver, ground corn,
animal fat, corn gluten meal, powdered cellulose

Protein 12.70%   **Fat** 8.50%   **Fiber** .50%   **Moisture** 72.5%
Magnesium .02%   **Calories** 221 per 5 1/2 oz. can
Urine pH 6.0–6.3   **Feeding:** as per your veterinarian's
directions

Prescription Diet® Health Blend Kitten® (dry)
Ingredients: poultry by-product meal, ground corn, animal fat
(preserved with BHA, propyl gallate and citric acid), corn
gluten meal, brewer's rice, chicken liver digest

Protein 33.43%   **Fat** 21.94%   **Fiber** 2.43%
Magnesium 0.76%   **Calories** 498 Kcal per 8 oz. cup
Feeding: as per veterinarian's directions

Prescription Diet® Health Blend Kitten® (canned)
Ingredients: water, liver, chicken, ground corn, poultry by-
product meal, meat by-products

Protein 13%   **Fat** 10.24%   **Fiber** .2%   **Magnesium** .02%
Calories 224 Kcal per 15 oz. can   **Urine pH** 6.1–6.4
Feeding: as per veterinarian's directions

Prescription Diet® Health Blend Adult® (dry)
Ingredients: ground corn, poultry by-product meal, corn
gluten meal, animal fat (preserved with BHA, propyl gallate
and citric acid), brewer's rice, chicken liver digest

Protein 30.29%   **Fat** 10.75%   **Fiber** 1.75%
Magnesium .086%   **Urine pH** 6.1–6.4
Calories 509 per cup   **Feeding:** 10-pound cat: 1/2 cup daily

Prescription Diet® Health Blend Geriatric® (canned)
product is new, information not yet available as this book went
to press

Comments: *Hills has supported veterinary nutrition growth for decades,
with studies conducted at major universities. While their formulas are
fixed formulas, I wish they had less cereal in their dry foods.*

IAMS CAT FOOD®
The Iams Company
Lewisburg, Ohio 45338
1-800-525-4267

Formulations: Iams Kitten Food, Iams Cat Food, Iams Less Active for Cats, Iams Natural Lamb & Rice, Iams canned cat food (Ocean Fish Formula, Whitefish Formula, Beef and Liver Formula, Chicken Formula, Turkey Formula), Eukanuba Veterinary Diets through veterinarian's prescription only

Iams Kitten Food (dry)—AAFCO-tested for growth
Ingredients: chicken by-products meal, chicken, rice, flour, ground corn, chicken fat (preserved with BHA), dried egg product, beet pulp, poultry digest, fish meal

Protein 34%   **Fat** 22%   **Fiber** 3%   **Ash** 7%
Magnesium .095%   **Moisture** 10%   **Calories** 468 per cup
Urine pH 6.1–6.4   **Feeding:** 1–3-pound kitten, approx 1/4 cup; 7–9-pound kitten, 3/4–2 1/4 cup

Iams Cat Food (dry)—AAFCO-tested for all life stages
Ingredients: chicken by-products meal, chicken, rice flour, ground corn, chicken fat (preserved with BHA), beet pulp, dried egg product, poultry digest, fish meal, brewer's dried yeast

Protein 32%   **Fat** 21%   **Fiber** 3%   **Ash** 6.5%
Magnesium .095%   **Moisture** 10%   **Calories** 432 per cup
Urine pH 6.1–6.4   **Feeding:** 10-pound cat: 1/3–1/2 cup daily

Iams Less Active Cat Food (dry)—AAFCO-tested for all life stages
Ingredients: chicken, chicken by-products meal, rice flour, ground corn, beet pulp, dried egg product, poultry digest, fish meal, chicken fat (preserved with BHA), brewer's dried yeast

Protein 28%   **Fat** 14%   **Fiber** 3%   **Ash** 6.5%
Magnesium .095%   **Moisture** 10%   **Calories** 348 per cup
Urine pH 6.1–6.4   **Feeding:** For weight maintenance of a 6–8-pound cat, feed 1/3–1/2 cup daily; for weight reduction of a 6–8-pound cat, feed 1/4–1/3 cup

Iams Lamb & Rice Cat Food (dry)—AAFCO-tested for all life stages

Ingredients: lamb, rice flour, chicken by-products meal, ground corn, animal fat (preserved with mixed tocopherols), fish meal, dried egg product, beet pulp, poultry digest

Protein 32%   Fat 21%   Fiber 3.0%   Ash 7.8%
Magnesium .095%   Moisture 78%   Calories 460 per cup
Urine pH 6.1–6.4   Feeding: 1/4 cup twice daily or free feed

Iams Beef Formula Cat Food (canned)—AAFCO-tested for all life stages

Ingredients: beef liver, water, beef, egg, chicken fat, rice flour

Protein 10%   Fat 6%   Fiber 1%   Ash 1.9%
Magnesium .025%   Moisture 78%
Calories 117 per 3 oz. can   Feeding: two 3-oz. cans daily

Iams Less Active for Cats (canned)—AAFCO-tested for maintenance

Varieties: Fish and Rice Formula, Chicken and Rice Formula

Iams Less Active for Cats (Fish and Rice Formula) (canned)

Ingredients: water, whitefish, beef, beef liver, beef by-products, rice flour, chicken by-products, dried egg product, fish meal

Protein 10%   Fat 3.5%   Fiber 1%   Ash 1.9%
Moisture 78%   Magnesium .02%   Calories 91 per 3 oz. can
Urine pH 6.1–6.4   Feeding: two 3-oz. cans daily

Eukanuba Veterinary Diets Response Formula LB/Feline (canned)—AAFCO-tested for maintenance

Protein 9%   Fat 6%   Ash less than 1.9%
Magnesium less than .015%   Moisture 78%
Urine pH 6.0–6.4

Formulated for cats with skin and coat or intestinal problems. See your veterinarian for details.

Eukanuba Veterinary Diets Restricted Calorie TM/Feline (dry)—AAFCO-tested for maintenance

Protein 32%   Fat 8%   Ash 7%   Magnesium .1%
Moisture 10%   Urine pH 6.0–6.4

Formulated for weight loss or maintenance. See your veterinarian for details.

Comments: A private company, Iams is truly dedicated to learning more about feline nutrition and makes quality foods. They have many nutritionists and veterinarians studying dogs and cats of all breeds and types.

OLD MOTHER HUBBARD®

Old Mother Hubbard Feed Company
P.O. Box 1719
Lowell, Massachusetts 01853-1719
1-800-225-0904

Old Mother Hubbard (canned)—AAFCO-tested for adults, 13 varieties

Varieties: Liver and Egg Dinner, Liver Dinner, Beef, Cheese and Egg Dinner, Beef and Chicken Dinner, Liver Dinner, Beef Dinner, Beef and Liver Dinner, Beef and Salmon Dinner, Beef and Tuna Dinner, Ocean Fish Dinner, just to name a few

Calories vary on flavor from 215–306

Urine pH approx 6.18

Old Mother Hubbard (canned) Beef and Tuna Dinner

Ingredients: beef by-products, beef broth, chicken by-products, beef, chicken, liver, ocean fish, tuna, salmon, wheat flour, dried egg product, bone meal, guar gum

Protein 9%   **Fat** 6.50%   **Fiber** 1%   **Ash** 1.8%
Moisture 78%   **Magnesium** .025%

Old Mother Hubbard Premium Nutrition Cat Food (dry)— AAFCO-tested for adults

Ingredients: poultry meal, rice flour, ground corn, corn gluten meal, dried egg product, animal fat (preserved with mixed tocopherols and citric acid), fish meal, tuna digest

Protein 31%   **Fat** 14%   **Fiber** 3.0%   **Ash** 6.0%
Moisture 10.0%   **Magnesium** 0.1%
Urine pH not available

Comments: If you have a finicky cat, you are bound to find a flavor that will please him. I'd like to see this company fund feline nutritional studies and help us all learn more about nutrition for cats.

TRIUMPH®
Product of Canada
Packed for Triumph Pet Industries, Inc.
Hilburn, New York
1-800-331-5144

Triumph Canned Cat Food®—AAFCO-tested for adults, 6 oz.,
3 oz.

Varieties: Beef and Chicken, Beef, Liver and Bacon, Beef and Chicken Dinner, Beef and Salmon Dinner, Turkey Dinner, to name a few.

Ash varies from 1.2–1.4% **Magnesium** .02%
Urine pH ranges 6.2–6.5
Calories ranges, depending on flavor.

Turkey

Ingredients: water sufficient for processing, meat by-products, turkey, beef, poultry by-products, poultry giblets, whole egg, guar gum, carrageenin, vitamin E supplement . . .

Protein 10.5% **Fat** 6% **Fiber** 1% **Ash** 1.4%
Moisture 78% **Magnesium** .02%

Triumph for Kittens®—AAFCO-tested for all stages of life

Varieties: Turkey Dinner, Sea Food Dinner

Seafood

Ingredients: ocean fish, meat by-products, water sufficient for processing, poultry by-products, liver, dry skimmed milk, rice flour, guar gum . . .

Protein 12% **Fat** 6% **Fiber** 1% **Ash** 2.5%
Moisture 78% **Magnesium** .02%
Calories 90 per 3 oz. can, 180 per 6 oz. can
Urine pH no data **Feeding:** Feed your kitten what it will eat in two or three feedings a day

Triumph Dry for Kittens®—"All-natural" will be available next
year

Triumph Premium Adult Maintenance Dry Cat Food®—AAFCO-
tested for adults

Ingredients: poultry meal, corn gluten meal, ground corn, poultry fat (preserved with BHA), ground rice, wheat flour, dried whole egg, brewer's dried yeast, dried chicken digest, phosphoric acid . . .

Protein 32%   **Fat** 20%   **Fiber** 2.5%   **Ash** 6%
Moisture 10%   **Magnesium** .1%   **Calories** 540 per cup
Urine pH 5.9–6.2

Will have a natural product next year.
Will have a natural lite product next year as well.

Triumph Lite Dinner for Cats®—AAFCO-tested for adults
Varieties: Turkey now, Seafood available next year

Turkey
Ingredients: water, meat by-products, turkey, beef liver, poultry giblets, poultry by-products . . .

Protein 11%   **Fat** 4%   **Fiber** 1.5%   **Moisture** 78%
Ash 1.4%   **Magnesium** .02%   **Urine pH** 6.2–6.5
Calories 3 oz. can 80, 6 oz. can 160, 14 oz. can 373
Feeding: 6 oz. can daily or two 3-oz. cans (6 oz. per 8-pound cat)

Has 20% less calories than Triumph canned

Protein 11%   **Fat** 6.0%   **Fiber** 1%   **Ash** 1.4%
Moisture 78%   **Magnesium** .02%
Calories 6 oz. can 185, 14 oz. can 433   **Urine pH** 6.2–6.5

Felo Diet for cats®—AAFCO-tested for adults (canned 3 oz., 6 oz., 14 oz.)
Ingredients: beef, water sufficient for processing, meat by-products, poultry by-products, liver, chicken, whole egg, guar gum . . .

Protein 11%   **Fat** 6.0%   **Fiber** 1%   **Ash** 1.4%
Moisture 78%   **Magnesium** .02%
Calories 3 oz. can 93, 6 oz. 185, 14 oz. 433   **Urine Ph** 6.2–6.5
Feeding: 6 oz. daily for average 6–8-pound cat

Felo Diet for Cats Dry—AAFCO-tested for adults
Ingredients: poultry meal, ground brewer's rice, poultry fat (preserved with BHA and citric acid), ground yellow corn, corn gluten meal, dried whole egg, brewer's dried yeast, phosphoric acid, poultry digest . . .

Protein 32%   **Fat** 20%   **Fiber** 2.0%   **Ash** 5.0%
Moisture 10%   **Magnesium** .08%   **Calories** 583 per cup
Urine pH 6.2–6.5   **Feeding:** an average cat, about 1/2 cup (8 oz.) daily

Comments: I find this canned food to be one of the most palatable on the market.

PRECISE CAT FOOD®

Precise Pet Products
P.O. Box 63009
Nacogdoches, Texas 75963
1-800-446-7148

Feline Foundation Formula® (dry)—AAFCO-tested for adults and growth

Ingredients: chicken meal, ground yellow corn, ground brown rice, corn gluten meal, poultry fat (preserved with d-alpha-tocopherol and ascorbyl palmitate), whole wheat flour, soybean meal, poultry digest, dried cheese, dried whey . . .

Protein 30%   **Fat** 16%   **Fiber** 3%   **Ash** 5.20%
Moisture 10%   **Magnesium** .12%
Calories 477 per cup   **Urine pH** 6.3

Feline Light Formula® (dry)—AAFCO-tested for adults

Ingredients: chicken meal, ground brown rice, whole wheat flour, ground yellow corn, corn gluten meal, wheat bran, soybean meal, poultry fat (preserved with d-alpha-tocopherol and ascorbyl palmitate), poultry digest, dried whey . . .

Protein 18%   **Fat** 10%   **Fiber** 4%   **Ash** 5%
Magnesium .12%   **Moisture** 10%   **Calories** 442 per cup
Urine pH 6.3

Comments: A relative newcomer to the alternative pet foods, they are pesticide-free. The chelated minerals and use of Ester C make them a wholesome food.

PRO PLAN CAT FOODS®

Pro-visions
Pet Specialty Enterprises
Division of Ralston Purina
Saint Louis, Mo 63188
1-800-688 PETS

Pro Plan, The Growth Plan (dry)—AAFCO-tested for growth
   Ingredients: chicken, corn gluten meal, brewer's rice, poultry by-products meal, ground yellow corn, animal fat (preserved with mixed tocopherols), phosphoric acid

   Protein 33%   **Fat** 20%   **Fiber** 3.0%   **Moisture** 12%
   Magnesium .10%   **Urine pH** not available
   Calories 452 per cup

Pro Plan, The Adult Plan (dry)—AAFCO-tested for adults
   Ingredients: corn gluten meal, chicken, wheat flour, brewer's rice, ground yellow corn, animal fat (preserved with mixed tocopherols), egg product

   Protein 31%   **Fat** 14%   **Fiber** 2.0%   **Ash** 6.2%
   Moisture 10%   **Magnesium** .06%   **Urine pH** not available
   Calories 435 per cup

Pro Plan Natural Turkey Barley Formula (dry)—AAFCO-tested for adults
   Ingredients: turkey, barley, corn gluten meal, corn turkey meal, animal fat preserved with mixed tocopherols, egg product, dried brewer's yeast, dried whey, phosphoric acid

   Protein 31%   **Fat** 14%   **Fiber** 2.0%   **Ash** 6.0%
   Moisture 12%   **Magnesium** .10%   **Urine pH** not available
   Calories 409 per cup

Pro Plan, The Lite Plan (dry))—AAFCO-tested for adults
   Ingredients: corn gluten meal, brewer's rice, chicken, ground yellow corn, wheat flour, corn bran, animal fat (preserved with mixed tocopherols), poultry by-products meal, phosphoric acid

   Protein 32%   **Fat** 6.5%   **Fiber** 5.0%   **Ash** 6.0%
   Magnesium .068%   **Moisture** 12%
   Calories 322 per 8 oz. cup   **Urine pH** not available

Purina Veterinarian Only®
Purina CNM—clinical nutrition management products

UR Formula—Feline Diet (dry)—for management of FLUTD
   Ingredients: corn gluten meal, beef, brewer's rice, wheat flour, ground yellow corn, beef tallow (preserved with mixed tocopherols), egg product, soy bean flour . . .

Protein 32.36%   **Fat** 10.60%   **Fiber** 1.36%   **Ash** 5.38%
Magnesium .07%   **Calories** 366 per 8 oz. cup
Urine pH 6.1

UR Formula—Feline Diet (canned)
Ingredients: beef, water, liver, meat by-product, beef tallow
(preserved with mixed tocopherols), brewer's rice, oat
groats . . .

Protein 12.12%   **Fat** 10.70%   **Fiber** .03%   **Ash** 1.65%
Moisture 70.71%   **Magnesium** .01%
Calories 217 per 5-1/2 oz. can   **Urine pH** 6.1

OM Formula—Feline Diet (dry)—for management of obesity
Ingredients: corn gluten meal, oat fiber, brewer's rice, poultry
by-product meal, soybean hulls, dried animal digest,
phosphoric acid . . .

Protein 32.20%   **Fat** 7.10%   **Fiber** 10.60%   **Ash** 7.01%
Moisture 7.57%   **Magnesium** .09%   **Calories** 283 per cup
Urine pH not available

*Comments: Pro Plan and the veterinary products certainly are a
professional alternative food, and good at that. I'd rather see
chicken fat than tallow, however.*

NUTRA MAX®
Nutra Products Inc.
445 Wilson Way
City of Industry, California 91744
1-800-833-5330

Max Cat Adult (dry)—AAFCO-tested for adults
Ingredients: chicken meal, corn gluten meal, wheat flour,
ground rice, poultry fat (preserved with ethoxyquin), ground
whole wheat, lamb meal, rice bran, dried whole egg, dried
brewer's yeast, natural flavors

Protein 32%   **Fat** 18%   **Fiber** 2.0%   **Ash** 6.50%
Magnesium 0.10%   **Calories** 435 per cup   **Urine pH** 6.0–6.4
Feeding: 10-pound cat: 1/2–2/3 cup

Max Cat Lite Food (dry)—AAFCO-tested for adults
Ingredients: chicken meal, ground rice, corn gluten meal,
wheat flour, rice bran, dried whole egg, poultry fat (preserved

with ethoxyquin), natural flavorings, lamb meal, sunflower, canola oils

Protein 32%   **Fat** 10%   **Fiber** 6.0%   **Ash** 6.50%
Magnesium .01%   **Calories** 359 per cup   **Urine pH** 6.0–6.4
Feeding: 10-pound cat: 1/2–2/3 cup for maintenance, 1/3–1/2 cup for weight reduction

Max Cat Kitten (dry)—AAFCO-tested for growth
Ingredients: chicken meal, corn gluten meal, wheat flour, ground rice, poultry fat (preserved with ethoxyquin), ground whole wheat, lamb meal, rice bran, dried whole egg

Protein 34%   **Fat** 20%   **Fiber** 3.0%   **Ash** 7.0%
Magnesium .10%   **Urine pH** not available   **Calories** 461/cup

Max Cat (canned)—AAFCO-tested for adults
Varieties: Original Formula, Chicken & Liver Formula, Turkey & Giblets, Ocean Fish Formula

Max Cat Original Formula
Ingredients: chicken broth, lamb liver, mackerel, ground rice, lamb, whole egg

Protein 10%   **Fat** 5%   **Fiber** 1.0%   **Ash** 2.0%
Moisture 78%   **Magnesium** .022%   **Urine pH** not available
Calories 169.1 per can (5.5 oz.)

Max Cat Lite (canned)—AAFCO-tested for adults
Varieties: Chicken & Ocean Fish, Turkey & Chicken, Chicken & Lamb

Max Cat Lite, Original Formula
Ingredients: chicken broth, chicken, chicken liver, mackerel, chicken giblets, turkey, lamb, ground rice, wheat gluten, potatoes, carrots, whole egg, guar gum and carrageenin, wheat bran

Protein 9.5%   **Fat** 3.0%   **Fiber** 3.0%   **Ash** 2.5%
Moisture 78%   **Magnesium** .025%   **Urine pH** not available

NATURAL CHOICE ADULT CAT FOOD®

Natural Choice Adult Cat Food (canned)—AAFCO-tested for adults
Varieties: Chicken Formula, Lamb & Rice Formula

Natural Choice Adult Cat Food Chicken Formula
Ingredients: chicken broth, chicken, chicken liver, turkey, mackerel, lamb, ground rice, wheat gluten, whole egg, wheat bran, guar gum and carrageenin, DL methionine, taurine, onion powder, garlic powder

Protein 10%   **Fat** 5%   **Fiber** 1.0%   **Ash** 1.5%
Moisture 78%   **Urine pH** 6.1–6.5
Calories 165.48 per 5.5 oz. can

Natural Choice Adult Cat Food (dry)—AAFCO-tested for adults
Ingredients: chicken meal, ground rice, rice gluten meal, whole dried egg, rice flour, poultry fat preserved with vitamin E, rice bran, lamb meal, dried brewer's yeast

Protein 30%   **Fat** 14%   **Fiber** 2.0%   **Ash** 6.50%
Magnesium .10%   **Urine pH** 6.1–6.5   **Calories** 402 per cup

Comments: I'd like to see less cereals in their dry food, with the elimination of wheat. Their food is extremely palatable. I'd like to see them fund feline nutrition studies and put their food through some more testing.

NATURES RECIPE®
Natures Recipe Pet Foods
Corona, CA 91720
1-800-843-4008

Natures Recipe Feline Diet (canned)—AAFCO-tested for all life stages
Varieties: Chicken Formula, Beef Formula, Rabbit Formula

Natures Recipe Feline Diet, Rabbit Formula
Ingredients: rabbit by-products, water, rabbit, brown rice, canola oil

Protein 10%   **Fat** 4.5%   **Fiber** 2.0%   **Ash** 2.5%
Moisture 78%   **Magnesium** .02%   **Calories** 156 per cup
Urine pH 6.0–6.5

Natures Recipe Lite (dry)—AAFCO-tested for adults
Ingredients: chicken meal, ground whole brown rice, pearled barley, soybean meal, lamb meal, animal digest, lamb fat (preserved with tocopherols), lamb meal, tomato pumice, lamb meal

Protein 28%   **Fat** 8.0%   **Fiber** 9.0%   **Ash** 6.0%
Moisture 10%   **Magnesium** .10%   **Urine pH** 6.1–6.5
Calories 411 per cup   **Feeding:** adult cat, 3/4–1 cup daily

Natures Recipe Maintenance Feline Diet (dry)—AAFCO-tested for all life stages

Ingredients: chicken meal, ground whole brown rice, cracked pearl barley, animal digest, soy bean meal, lamb fat (preserved with tocopherols and ascorbic acid), lamb meal, dried liver meal, tomatoes pumice, canola oil

Protein 32%   **Fat** 15%   **Fiber** 4.0%   **Ash** 6.0%
Moisture 10%   **Magnesium** .09%   **Urine pH** 6.0–6.5
Calories 482 per 4 oz. cup   **Feeding:** adult cats, 3/4–1 cup daily; kittens, free choice

Innovative Veterinary Diets (dry)—AAFCO-tested for all life stages

sold by veterinarians only

Formulations: Duck & Potato, Lamb & Potato, Venison & Potato

Innovative Veterinary Diets (dry) Duck & Potato

Ingredients: potato, duck, duck meal, duck fat (preserved with tocopherols and ascorbic acid), canola oil, duck digest

Protein 30%   **Fat** 12%   **Fiber** 4.5%   **Ash** 6.0%
Moisture 10.0%   **Magnesium** .05%
Urine pH not available

Innovative Veterinary Diets (canned) Lamb & Potato

Ingredients: water sufficient for processing, lamb, lamb by-products, lamb liver, potato, canola oil

Protein 9.0%   **Fat** 5.5%   **Fiber** 1.5%   **Ash** 1.8%
Moisture 78%   **Urine pH** not available

Comments: *This company seems to be doing everything right. Their products, both veterinary and direct consumer, can help allergic or sensitive cats.*

FRISKIES®
Friskies Pet Care Company
Glendale, California
Carnation
1-800-933-0991

Friskies Fancy Feast (canned)—AAFCO-tested for all life stages, 3 oz. cans
Varieties: Ocean Feast, Tender Liver & Chicken Feast, Tender Beef Feast, Salmon & Chicken Feast, Chicken Hearts & Liver Feast, Turkey Feast, Tuna & Mackerel Feast and more.

Formulas vary according to mouth size: regular, minced, sliced, and flaked

Friskies Fancy Feast (canned) Tuna & Mackerel Feast
Ingredients: sufficient water for processing, tuna, fish, chicken, turkey, wheat gluten, mackerel, meat by-products, soy flour, soy protein concentrate, natural and artificial flavors, sodium nitrite

Protein 14.0% **Fat** 3.0% **Fiber** 1.0% **Ash** 3.5%
Moisture 78.0% **Magnesium** .03% **Urine pH** 6.0–6.4
Feeding: 10-pound cat, 8.9 oz. daily (almost three 3-oz. cans)

Friskies Fancy Feast Gourmet Dry Cat Food, Turkey & Giblets— AAFCOT-tested for all life stages
Ingredients: brewer's rice, poultry by-products meal, corn gluten meal, digest containing poultry by-products, animal fat (preserved with BHA), ground wheat, ground yellow corn, color, yellow #5

Protein 30% **Fat** 15% **Fiber** 4.5% **Ash** 5.9%
Moisture 12% **Magnesium** .85% **Calories** 385 per cup
Feeding: 8–12-pound cat, 3/4–1 cup daily

Friskies Premium Chef's Blend—Four-Flavor Dry Cat Food
Ingredients: ground yellow corn, digest (chicken by-products, fish and fish by-products), poultry by-products meal, corn gluten meal, soybean meal, fish meal, phosphoric acid, animal fat (preserved with BHA), shrimp meal, salt, natural and artificial flavors

Protein 30% **Fat** 8.0% **Fiber** 4.5% **Moisture** 12.0%
Ash 6.4% **Magnesium** .13% **Calories** 348 per cup
Urine pH not available **Feeding:** 10-pound cat, 3/4 cup daily

Friskies Senior (canned)—AAFCO-tested for adults
    Varieties: Tender Cuts, Chicken & Tuna in Gravy, Savory Beef
    & Gravy, Pacific Salmon in Sauce, Turkey & Giblets in Gravy

Friskies Senior (canned) Tender Cuts Chicken & Tuna Dinner
    Ingredients: water sufficient for processing, chicken, liver,
    meat by-products, wheat gluten, turkey, modified food starch,
    tuna, soy flour, natural and artificial flavors, brewer's rice, soy
    protein concentrate, taurine
    Protein 9.0%   **Fat** 3.5%   **Fiber** 1.0%   **Moisture** 78.0%
    Ash 2.5%   **Magnesium** .02%   **Urine pH** not available
    Feeding: 1 can per 5 lbs., 25% less for cats 7 years and older

*Friskies Special Diet for Adult Cats (dry)—AAFCO-tested for
adults*
    Ingredients: ground yellow corn, corn gluten meal, digest
    (chicken by-products, phosphoric acid), poultry by-products
    meal, animal fat (preserved with BHA)
    Protein 29%   **Fat** 14.0%   **Fiber** 2.5%   **Ash** 6.5%
    Magnesium .085%   **Urine pH** not available
    Feeding: 10-pound cat, 3/4–1 1/4 cup

    Formulated for cats at risk of FLUTD

    Comments: *While I'm satisfied with Friskies' testing and thank
    them for their nutritional studies, I'd like to see less cereal in their
    dry foods and removal of sodium nitrite in their canned foods. Their
    canned foods are relatively expensive if you look at the quantity you
    need to feed.*

PURINA®
    Ralston Purina
    St. Louis, Missouri 63164
    1-800-7-purina

Tender Vittles—AAFCO-tested for adults
    Varieties: Sea Food Dinner, Chicken Dinner, Beef Dinner, Tuna
    Dinner

Tender Vittles, Tuna Dinner
    Ingredients: water for processing, poultry by-products meal,
    corn gluten meal, ground yellow corn, soy bean meal, wheat
    flour, chicken, animal fat (preserved with BHA), tuna meal,

phosphoric acid, brewer's dried yeast, fumaric acid, salt, ascorbic acid (a preservative), added color

Protein 24% **Fat** 8.5% **Fiber** 3.5% **Moisture** 39%
Calories 120 per package **Urine pH** not available
Feeding: 6–8-pound cat, 2 1/2 pouches daily

Purina Cat Chow (dry) original formula—AAFCO-tested for all life stages

Ingredients: ground yellow corn, corn gluten meal, soy bean meal, poultry by-products meal, animal fat (preserved with BHA), fish meal, meat and bone meal, ground wheat

Protein 31.5% **Fat** 8.0% **Fiber** 4.5% **Moisture** 12%
Magnesium .13% **Calories** 371 per 8 oz. cup
Urine pH not available **Feeding:** 10–14-pound cat, 1 1/4 cup daily

Purina Kitten Chow (dry)—AAFCO-tested for all life stages
Varieties: Dairy Formula, Original

Purina Kitten Chow, Dairy Formula
Ingredients: poultry by-products meal, soybean meal, ground yellow corn, corn gluten meal, ground wheat, brewer's rice, whey, animal fat (preserved with BHA), phosphoric acid

Protein 35% **Fat** 8.5% **Fiber** 4% **Moisture** 12%
Magnesium .14% **Calories** 345 per cup **Urine pH** not available
Feeding: 7 weeks to 6 months, 1-1 1/3 cup daily

Purina Meow Mix (dry)—AAFCO-tested for all life stages
Ingredients: ground yellow corn, corn gluten meal, chicken by-products meal, soy bean meal, beef tallow (preserved with mixed tocopherols), turkey by-products meal, salmon meal, dried animal digest, phosphoric acid

Protein 31.0% **Fat** 8.0% **Fiber** 4.0% **Moisture** 12%
Magnesium .13% **Urine pH** not available **Calories** 371/cup

Purina canned—AAFCO-tested for adults
Varieties (18+): Beef Platter, Turkey & Chicken Dinner, Tender Beef Dinner, Turkey & Giblets Dinner, Tuna Dinner, Tuna & Egg, Tender Beef Dinner

Purina Turkey & Giblets Dinner
Ingredients: water for processing, meat by-products, turkey giblets, turkey, rice

Protein 10%   **Fat** 4.0%   **Fiber** 1.0%   **Ash** 3.0%
Moisture 78%   **Magnesium** .05%   **Calories** 225 per can
Feeding: one can daily

Comments: While I am certain of Purina's formulations and testing, I'd like to see more meat and less cereal. I only recommend Tender Vittles for cats with diarrhea, short-term only. I applaud Purina's support of veterinary medicine and all the studies they have funded.

9 LIVES CAT FOOD®
Heinz pet products
Newport, Kentucky 41071
1-800-252-7022

9 Lives Plus Canned Cat Food—AAFCO-tested for all life stages
Varieties (30+): Turkey & Giblets, Tuna & Cheese, Chicken & Beef Dinner, Super Supper, Tuna & Egg Dinner, Ocean Whitefish Dinner, Sliced Beef & Gravy

There are two mouth sizes: Ground and flaked, sliced and shredded

9 Lives Plus Canned Cat Food—general analysis
Ingredients: water sufficient to process, veal, meat by-products, poultry by-products, wheat flour, modified starch, high-fructose corn syrup, whey powder, soy protein concentrate, fish by-products, bone meal, salt, onion

Protein   10.2%   **Fat** 9.0%   **Ash** 2.6%   **Fiber** 1.3%
Magnesium .031%   **Calories** 38 Kcal/oz.
Urine pH not available
Feeding: 6–8-pound cat, one can twice daily

9 Lives Plus Care Low pH (dry)—AAFCO-tested for adults
Ingredients: ground yellow corn, corn gluten meal, poultry by-products meal, source of chicken and turkey flavors, ground wheat, animal digest, animal fat (preserved with BHA), meat and bone meal, natural and artificial flavors, red dye # 40

Protein 31.2% **Fat** 10.9% **Fiber** 1.6% **Ash** 6.3%
Moisture 8.5% **Magnesium** .090% **Urine pH** 6.01
Calories 100 per oz.

Helps maintain urinary tract health by reducing the pH

Amore Canned Cat Food—AAFCO-tested for all life stages
   Varieties (13 in all): meat based, poultry based, fish based;
   Chicken Hearts & Liver, Diced Veal & Gravy, Simmered Beef &
   Chicken, Beef Slices Entreé, Pacific White Fish & Shrimp, Sea
   Food Supreme, Savory Chicken & Tuna, Turkey & Giblets

Amore Natural (canned), Chicken Hearts & Liver Entreé for cats
   Ingredients: water sufficient to process, chicken hearts,
   chicken, liver, chicken by-products, wheat gluten, wheat flour

   Protein 10% **Fat** 2.0% **Fiber** 1.0% **Ash** 2.5%
   Moisture 78% **Magnesium** .018% **Urine pH** 6.2
   Calories 98 per can

   Comments: *While all the foods taste great, I'm not crazy about
   fructose, cereal content, and the artificial coloring in some of these
   foods.*

KAL KAN FOODS, INC.®
   Vernon, California 90058
   1-800-525-5273

*Whiskas Meat Food for Cats and Kittens (canned)—AAFCO-
tested for all life stages*   .
   Varieties (17+): Cat Fish, Chicken & Tuna, Kitty Stew, Pick of
   the Ocean, Meal Time, Bits of Beef

Whiskas Meat Food for Cats and Kittens, Bits of Beef
   Ingredients: meat by-products, poultry by-products, water,
   beef, liver, kidney, guar gum

   Protein 9.0% **Fat** 5.0% **Fiber** 1.5% **Magnesium** .018%
   Urine pH not available **Calories** 153 per can
   Feeding: 8-pound cat, 1 1/2 cans daily

Whiskas Dry Cat Food—AAFCO-tested for all stages of life
   Varieties: Original Crave Recipe, Poultry, Sea Food

Whiskas Dry Cat Food, Original Crave Recipe
Ingredients: ground yellow corn, chicken by-products meal, soy bean meal, ground wheat, poultry digest, meat, dried milk protein, tuna meal, animal fat (preserved with BHA, BHT)

Protein 30%   **Fat** 8.0%   **Fiber** 4.5%   **Moisture** 12.0%
Magnesium .12%   **Calories** 310 per 8 oz. cup   **Urine pH** not available
Feeding: kittens, 1/4–1 1/2 cups daily; adults 1/2–1 1/4 cups daily

Sheba Food for Cats (canned)—AAFCO-tested for all life stages
Varieties (9+): Gourmet Salmon & Aspic with Poultry lightly simmered in meat juices, Select Meaty Juices, Tender Beef in Meaty Juices

Sheba Food for Cats, Tender Beef in Meaty Juices
Ingredients: sufficient water for processing, beef by-products, meat by-products, liver, poultry by-products, beef, calcium carbonate, carrageenin, xanthan gum, guar gum, caramel coloring

Protein 8.0%   **Fat** 3.5%   **Fiber** 1.0%   **Ash** 3.0%
Moisture 82%   **Magnesium** .018%   **Calories** 76   **Urine pH** not available
Feeding: 8-pound cat, three trays

Waltham Formulas (dry or canned)—Available for growth, adult, senior, and lite

Waltham Formula Growth Diet for Cats (canned), Chicken Dinner—AAFCO-tested for growth
Ingredients: meat by-products, sufficient water for processing, chicken, chicken liver and heart, beef by-products, dried egg, dried cottage cheese, vegetable gums

Protein 11%   **Fat** 7.5%   **Fiber** 1.0%   **Ash** 2.0%
Magnesium .025%   **Calories** 185 Kcal/can   **Feeding:** 6–16 weeks of age, 3/4–1 1/2 cans daily; 16 weeks of age, 1 1/4 cans–2 cans daily

Waltham Formula Growth Diet for cats (dry)—AAFCO-tested for growth
Ingredients: chicken by-products meal, rice, ground corn, corn gluten meal, ground wheat, digest of poultry by-products,

animal fat (preserved with BHA), dried milk protein, brewer's yeast

Protein 32%   **Fat** 11%   **Fiber** 3.0%   **Moisture** 12%
Ash 7.0%   **Magnesium** .14%   **Calories** 185 Kcal per can
Feeding: 6–16 weeks, 3/4–1 1/2 cans daily; 16 weeks–36 weeks, 1 1/4–2 cans daily

Waltham Formula Adult Conditioning Diet for Cats (canned) Chicken & Rice—AAFCO-tested for adults

Ingredients: water sufficient for processing, chicken, chicken liver and heart, chicken by-products, brewer's rice, vegetable gums

Protein 9.0%   **Fat** 7.0%   **Fiber** 1.5%   **Moisture** 78%
Ash 2.0%   **Magnesium** .03%   **Calories** 180 Kcal per can
Urine pH not available

Waltham Formula Lite Diet for Cats (dry)—AAFCO-tested for adults

Ingredients: ground corn, corn gluten meal, chicken by-products meal, rice, wheat mill run, digest of poultry by-products, brewer's yeast, dried whole egg

Protein 27%   **Fat** 6%   **Fiber** 5%   **Moisture** 12.0%
Ash 5.5%   **Magnesium** .13%   **Calories** 225 Kcal per cup
Urine pH not available

Comments: Waltham and Kal Kan have been involved with pet nutrition for a long time and I thank them for all their help. I wish they would decrease the amount of cereal in some of their foods. While Sheba tastes great, note that your average cat requires 3 trays daily. That's a lot of food.

CHAPTER 5

········· ··········

Feeding for Fitness

········· ··········

Know Your Cat's Age

Knowing the human equivalent of your cat's age will give you a better understanding of your pet's nutritional needs.

When does a kitten become a cat? A lot sooner than most owners realize. Technically, kittens are kittens until they're a year old, but a female enters puberty somewhere between three and nine months of age and can come into heat as early as three and a half months! Males are a little slower. They become pubescent around the age of seven months.

Being aware that your eight-month-old kitten is the feline equivalent to a thirteen-year-old teenager makes the cat's high nutritional requirements a lot more comprehensible. Everyone realizes that a growing, active teenager needs more daily protein, fat, vitamins and minerals than the average forty-year-old office worker, and food quantity and supplements are adjusted accordingly. But not everyone realizes that this also holds true for cats. A six-year-old cat who's still being fed the same diet and quantity as an eight-month-old kitten is going to be one plump puss with mounting pounds of health problems. (See "The Dangers of Feline Obesity" in chapter 11.)

Also, as a cat ages, its sense of smell and taste decrease, often causing an older animal to refuse its usual food. Weight loss and accompanying nutrient depletion at this stage of a cat's life can be extremely dangerous to its health. Knowing what highly palatable, digestible foods and supplements are called for is essential (see "New Life for Your Beloved Older Cat" later in this chapter), as is knowing your cat's age.

The following comparisons are given to help guide you in providing appropriate and optimum nutrition throughout your pet's life. (All ages are in years, except where indicated.)

Cat's Age	Human Age Equivalents
6 months	10
8 months	13
1	15
2	24
4	32
6	40
8	48
10	56
12	64
14	72
16	80
18	88
20	96
21	100
22	104

Prime Meals for Pregnant Cats

Feed your queen like a queen and the results will be royally rewarding.

Taking care of kittens before they are born is more your job than the mother's. Professional breeders have known for years that the better nutritional and physical shape a queen (pregnant cat) is in, the healthier her litter will be. An overweight cat who becomes pregnant, for instance, is a high risk for delivery complications, including kitten deformities and fatalities.

Considering your pet is going to be pregnant for only a little more than two months (sixty-three to sixty-six days is the typical gestation period), paying extra attention to her diet for that short a time is a minor inconvenience that will pay both of you back with major rewards.

No doubt about it, a pregnant cat must be provided with a constant supply of necessary nutrients for the proper fetal development of her kittens. In fact, a recent study at Colorado State University proved conclusively that a queen's diet directly affects the growth and health of all her kittens' vital organs.

Nutrient Musts for Moms-to-Be

VITAMINS A AND D:
If insufficiently supplied, growing fetuses will draw minerals from the mother and could cause serious nutritional deficiency in the queen.

VITAMIN B COMPLEX:
Needed for prevention of neurological birth defects and for protecting the queen against debilitating effects of stress.

VITAMIN C:
Important for reducing pregnancy stress and strengthening the queen's immune system.

CALCIUM AND PHOSPHORUS:
Vital for protecting the queen from mineral deficiency and for enabling the production of nutritive milk; necessary for proper growth of kittens' bones and teeth and for preventing malformations.

COPPER, IODINE AND ZINC:
Inadequate amounts in diet can cause birth defects in kittens.

FOLIC ACID:
Vital for the development of the nervous system.

IRON:

Necessary for making red blood cells—for resistance to disease for both mother and kittens and for growth of kittens.

FATTY ACIDS:

Inadequate amount can create all types of skin and coat problems in the mother and stunt the growth of the newborns.

Meals Fit for a Queen

A pregnant cat should be fed two, or preferably three, times daily. Dividing her daily ration into three portions is easier on the digestive system and will make her more comfortable during this period.

During the first month of pregnancy her protein quality and quantity should be increased, but *not* her caloric intake. If you are not feeding quality food (my first choice), then you must add a "whole food" supplement to fortify her diet. The best supplements are bee pollen (Dr. Jane® Beezyme Formula 1), blue-green algae, brewer's yeast, or torula yeast. You can give her the liver treats between meals as long as you don't keep her from eating her own balanced cat food. Liver is not particularly fattening and has an abundance of nutrients. Liver, like all meat, is low in calcium; however, you don't have to worry about calcium, since all brand-named cat foods (alternative or supermarket) have enough calcium. As a matter of fact, adding a calcium supplement to your queen's diet is an absolute NO, but if you are a nervous mother and want to do something—give her some cottage cheese or yogurt as treats. Make sure the yogurt is low-fat, since we want her to keep in shape so that she doesn't get fat and have a problem with delivery.

During the second month of pregnancy, caloric needs are greater. Where a cat would ordinarily need 40 calories per pound of body weight daily, when pregnant she needs at least 50. I'd advise increasing your mommy-to-be's daily food intake during her second month by 25 to 75 percent, depending on her size and appetite. Add additional food to each of her meals; or better yet, feed her an alternative professional kitten food. You can leave dry kitten food down all day allowing her to nibble. Just make sure you give her the feel test weekly to make sure she is not gaining too much weight.

During this stressful period, an abundance of tender loving care and a little special mealtime catering now and then will be greatly appreciated by your pet—and can make you both feel terrific. The following are New-Life recipes formulated as healthy, occasional, "treat" meals for pregnant cats. Lactating and nursing queens require more food (depending on their size and the size of the litter, they can eat three to four times as much as they did before pregnancy), so these recipes should be doubled for them.

Breakfast Fit for a Queen

1 egg	1 teaspoon butter
1 teaspoon lactose-free milk	1–2 pieces crisp bacon
1/2 cup instant oatmeal	optional: 1/8 teaspoon bee pollen

Beat the egg and milk. Add oatmeal. Melt the butter in a frying pan, and cook the eggs. Add the bacon and bee pollen when the eggs are done (don't overcook them).

Luncheon Treat

1/4 lb. lean, chopped hamburger meat	pinch of salt
1/4 cup cooked, brown rice	1/8 teaspoon minced garlic
1 whole egg (shell included)	optional: 1/8 teaspoon fresh, chopped wheat grass or a chopped vegetable
1/8 teaspoon olive oil or bacon fat	

Sauté the garlic in the olive oil or bacon fat. Add the chopped hamburger meat and the cooked rice. Pour the egg onto the meat and remove everything from the flame. Take the egg shell and chop it into small pieces—powder it, if you can. Add the finely chopped or powdered egg shell to the meat—return it to the flame, and cook, stirring frequently, flattening the rice. Add the chopped wheat grass just before the meat is lightly brown. Do not overcook the meat! Serve once the meal becomes room temperature.

Breakfast Fit for a Queen

While this meal is not as balanced as I would like (and should be considered a snack or treat), it will give mother-to-be an excellent source of high biological value protein and arachidonic acid—both helpful for this time of her life.

Fish Dinner Fit for a Queen

Fish Dinner	
1 small sole, halibut, or cod fillet (no bones please)	1/8 teaspoon chopped parsley (fresh is best)
1/8 teaspoon olive oil	1/8 teaspoon parmesan cheese
1/8 teaspoon minced garlic	
Sauté garlic in olive oil. Add fish, parmesan cheese and parsley. Cook. Serve when room temperature.	

Healthy Snacks

- Cantaloupe balls, two or three daily. They're low in calories and high in Vitamin C and B.
- 1/8–1/4 cup chopped, canned clams—a great taurine source.
- One or two tablespoons of yogurt. It's a good source of calcium and vitamin K.
- Cooked (fresh or canned) asparagus spears. Cats enjoy playing with and nibbling on them, and they supply iron.
- Small pieces of tomato. Tomato supplies potassium, vitamin C, and selenium, which helps vitamin E work more effectively.
- One or two small squares of mild cheese. A great source of calcium and protein.
- 1/4 cup canned or raw peas. A fine source of vitamin A and fiber and fun for cats to bat around.
- Leftover cooked vegetables, eggs, meats and broth can be mixed into regular balanced meals, but should not amount to more than 25 percent of the cat's usual serving.

No-No Snacks

- Spicy luncheon meats
- Italian sausage or pepperoni
- Chili
- Chocolate, spinach or rhubarb. They contain oxalic acid, which can interfere with the proper absorption of needed calcium.
- Grains and cereals. These contain phytic acid, which can impair calcium absorption.
- Extremely fatty foods (such as greasy table scraps, tallow, lard) can cause digestive upsets and impair calcium absorption.

Pregnancy Cautions

- *Do* make sure your cat has a booster distemper vaccination before pregnancy.
- *Don't* overfeed your cat with meals or treats. In the last week or two of pregnancy, be particularly careful. This is when she needs the most protein, vitamins and minerals, and the least amount of pound-adding carbohydrates.
- *Do* feed her in a calm setting and don't pick her up after eating so she can fully digest.
- *Do* allow your cat normal exercise, but if she is used to outdoor athletics, such as jumping from tree branches to window ledges, I'd suggest grounding her once she's into her second month of pregnancy.
- *Do* give your cat supplemental vitamin C if she's not getting at least 100 mg daily.
- *Don't* supplement your pet's diet with multiple vitamin-mineral preparations without consulting your veterinarian. Dr. Jane® Beezyme will **not** disturb your cat's food formula. Supplementing an inadequate or imbalanced diet incorrectly can cause even more harmful imbalances. For optimal health, there is no substitute for a balanced and adequate diet.
- *Do* call your veterinarian if she doesn't seem well; such as not eating, lethargic or listless.

- *Don't* give your cat commercial worm medicine while she's pregnant. Consult your veterinarian for a safe treatment.
- *Do* avoid low-quality or generic dry foods, which often cause digestive upsets (diarrhea or vomiting) in pregnant queens and nursing cats, who have voracious appetites.
- *Don't* give any medications unless you consult your veterinarian.

Getting Kitty Started

Picking up nutritionally where Momma leaves off can keep your kitten fit for life.

There's nothing like a mother's milk, particularly colostrum (the first milk produced after birth), to give a kitten the best possible healthy start in life. Colostrum contains the queen's antibodies, along with quality nutrients, which are passed on to the kittens in the first three days of nursing, providing them with an immediate immune system to fight off the wide variety of possible kittenhood infections and diseases.

A healthy queen will produce ample milk for her kittens for four or five weeks. After that, the quantity of milk usually decreases and the kittens should be weaned gradually.

Smooth transition: When weaning a kitten, make the switch pleasant, nutritional and digestibly rewarding. (You wouldn't expect a baby to go directly from breast to burgers, so don't expect a kitten to go from mom's milk to Meow Mix® without a howl.) An intermediate stage called "mush" is what I've found to be most successful on all levels.

Mush Menus

Anytime after three and a half weeks, you can mix a little bit of Pablum with warm skim milk (or Pet Ag's KMR or Hill's Feline P/D mixed with water) and offer it to the kittens on your finger. The sooner they learn how to lap (instead of suck), the easier the transition to feeding from mom to meal bowl will be.

Dr. Jane's Two-to-One Kitty Slurpies

1/4 cup professional/alternative canned kitten food	1/8 cup skim milk, water or Pet Ag's KMR

Blend 1/4 cup canned, complete and nutritionally balanced kitten food with 1/8 cup milk, water or Pet Ag's KMR. The kitten food should be the same as that fed the mother. The mother's milk tastes like the kitten food and will help the transition. The consistency should be about that of junior baby food. Once your kitten accepts the mush, decrease the amount of liquid daily.

Around the age of six weeks, your kitten should be ready and eager for solid meals—canned or dry. But always keep fresh water available in a shallow bowl! Don't use Fido's deep water dish. A kitten could tumble in and drown.

Alternative Beginnings for Orphan Kittens

Use any professional weaning formula (such as Pet Ag or KMR), which can be obtained from your veterinarian or pet food store; or use my home recipe:

Dr. Jane's Weaning Formula

1 egg yolk	1 teaspoon brewer's or torula yeast or bee pollen per mixture
1 teaspoon Karo or maple syrup per mixture	A vitamin-mineral supplement (such as Dr. Jane® Beezyme, Pro Balance, F-Biotic)
1 tablespoon heavy cream	

Mix equal parts evaporated or whole milk mixed with boiled water. Mix well and keep refrigerated until needed. Warm before feeding. Temperature should be tepid.

Orphan formulas can be fed from baby-doll bottles, special bottles available from vets or pet stores, or plastic medicine droppers. Never feed a kitten on its back! Place the animal on its stomach on a towel on your lap. Open the kitten's mouth gently and then insert the dropper or nipple. Be sure the nipple opening is not clogged! Keep it at an angle that will allow milk to flow slowly, yet prevent air from being sucked in. Pulling back occasionally on the bottle or dropper will stimulate the kitten's sucking reflex. Burp after feeding just as you would a baby. The kitten's tummy should feel full but not bloated. Four feedings a day are often sufficient, but I prefer five—and I find that most kittens do, too. You have to get up during the night for feedings; at least twice when they are newly born.

After three weeks, try to get the kitten to lap the formula from your finger and then proceed to encourage "mush" food eating, as described above. Ask your veterinarian about supplementary pediatric vitamin and mineral drops. These are a wise investment for kittens who've been deprived of their mother's nutrients.

Older orphaned kittens can be started on a specialized kitten food, such as Hill's Feline P/D (available with a veterinarian's prescription) or Iams Kitten Food at your pet store.

Kitty Feeding Tips and Other Cautions

1. Don't start your kitten on human food! Once kitty takes a liking to it, other food will be ignored, and you'll find that you've created a finicky eater. Kittens grow incredibly fast, and a quality balanced diet is essential for optimum health. Treat table scraps as occasional treats—not meals!
2. Allow your kitten at least one hour after eating before handling, especially by children. (You wouldn't appreciate a piggyback ride on a full stomach, would you?)
3. Be sure the room your kitten or kittens are in is large enough for exercise and free from hazards, such as toxic cleansers, plants, paints, small ingestible objects and large pets. It should also be out of the main household traffic area.
4. Sunlight is vital to proper bone and muscle development of your kittens. They should get at least one hour of direct sunlight daily, if possible.
5. Warmth, no matter how much fur those little fluffs of fun have, is necessary. Kittens under five weeks of age without a momma to snuggle into should have an electric heating pad (it must be waterproof) or a heating lamp to keep them warm when sleep-

ing. There should always be enough space, however, for the kitten to move away from the heat when it wants to.

6. If you are feeding your kitten dry food, make sure it's high quality.

7. Kittens should not look like tiny teddy bears. A sleek, firm, muscular kitten is a healthier kitten and will be a much healthier cat. Avoid meeting their caloric requirements with foods that contain too much cereal filler. Protein provides the most effective, efficient energy during growth.

8. If you want to save time and money by preparing a two-day supply of "mush," store it in an airtight container in the refrigerator. When reserving, add a little hot water to bring it to room temperature or put the bowl in hot water (as you would a baby's bottle), until the chill is gone. This will enhance the aroma of the food, increase its digestibility and prevent gastrointestinal upsets that are caused by cold food.

9. Start by feeding four small meals a day. Letting your kitten get too hungry can cause him to eat too quickly, and more often than not, will result in the unwanted return of that meal to your floor. If you have to be away at work during this period, feed your kitten breakfast laced with about one-fourth teaspoon Karo, maple or pancake syrup. Whenever a large gap between meals is unavoidable, this will stave off hunger and serve as a helpful energy supplement, but it is not advised as a regular practice. Feed the next meal when you come home and another meal before bedtime. If your kitten is able to chew dry food, leave that down—along with fresh water—and forgo the syrup.

10. At around three months of age, three meals daily (of approximately three ounces of quality food at each meal), should fill the needs of most growing kittens.

11. Don't leave food down for more than 10 to 20 minutes.

12. Don't add bone meal to your kitten's food. It could upset the proper calcium/phosphorus ratio.

13. Kittens should not be taken from their mother until they are at least six weeks old.

14. Vaccinations for distemper should be given when kittens are between six and eight weeks of age. Ask your veterinarian for the vaccination schedule.

Shaping Up a Stray the Right Way

How to turn a scraggly stray into a super cat

When a stray comes into your life, so can a host of problems, but so can some of the most loving rewards imaginable. Whether you selected the cat from an animal shelter or found it hungry, alone, and looking much like a moth-eaten muff someone tossed in an alley, the moment you bring it home you can begin rectifying its unhappy past and shaping it up for a happy, healthy, and revitalized, new life.

A Safe Start

If you have other pets at home, don't rush introductions. The wisest thing to do is isolate your new addition for at least a day before you take it to the vet for a thorough, professional check-up, which is essential even if you got the cat from an animal shelter. (If the poor cat is obviously in distress, then, of course, take it to a veterinarian immediately.) There are several important reasons for this:

- The cat might be harboring a communicable disease.
- You will have a chance to get acquainted and observe the cat, without dealing with the probable jealousy of other pets and the likely intimidation of your new arrival.
- You'll be able to supply your vet with important diagnostic information by providing a stool sample and reporting any unusual behavior or eating habits.
- If your new pet has any existing health problems or conditions, prompt medical treatment and advice can prevent a lot of heartache. Knowledge of the problems will also allow you to plan a diet that can be tailored specifically to provide your foundling with optimal health. (See chapter 11 for nutritional treatments of common ailments.)
- Put a scented powder or cologne on your "new" cat as soon as you bring it into the house, as well as on your existing one(s). That way everyone smells the same; continue for one week.

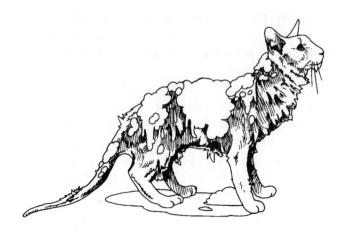

Important Don'ts

Don't give your stray a bath before it has been examined and you've asked the vet's approval. If the cat is in poor health, and chances are that it is, a bath could be extremely dangerous at this time and could cause a fatal case of pneumonia. I'd suggest wiping any dirt or excrement off with a warm, damp cloth, then toweling those areas dry immediately. Herbal pet wipes can clean and get rid of fleas! No dryers please!

Don't feed more than a small amount of food at first, no matter how hungry the little guy looks. If the cat has worms (a more than likely possibility), a sudden ingestion of food can cause mayhem in the poor creature's gastrointestinal tract and possibly its stool. Wait at least two hours after the cat has eaten before offering another small meal.

First Feedings

Assuming your new family member has no serious problems, starting off with my New-Life Diet is ideal for rapid recuperation from any previous dietary deficiencies, and the best immunity insurance possible for continuous well-being.

Not knowing what the cat has been used to eating can sometimes make starting a new feeding regime a tricky business. Cats, even hungry ones, can have very definite preferences in food texture and taste, and if addicted to one particular kind, they may refuse all others at first.

A change in environment, even if it's for the better, is a stress-inducing situation for a cat, commonly causing it to refuse all food. This might last for a day, even two. Don't be discouraged, and whatever you do, don't let your new cat train you!

NOTE: A food refusal that continues for more than two days warrants veterinary consultation.

Adoptive parents of strays are particularly vulnerable to falling into a "You don't like that? Well, how about this?" syndrome. The result, as I've seen many times, is bewildered owners who can't understand why, after waiting hand and paws upon their pets, their animals look (and are) in such sad shape.

You're Bigger and Smarter: Cats, much like children, might know what they like, but what they like is not always what's good for them. If you truly love your pet, the best way to show it is by giving it the gift of fitness through proper feeding.

The New-Life Healthy Start Diet for Strays

This diet is designed for an average 8-pound cat or one who should weigh that much, give or take a couple of pounds. For the special needs of pregnant and lactating cats, growing kittens, diabetic, geriatric, obese cats, and others with exceptional nutrient requirements or restrictions, consult the index for individual sections.

1. Begin by weighing your cat. If ribs and spine are visible, your cat needs a higher daily caloric intake than indicated in chapter 3; if excess fat is present along the abdomen and you can't feel the cat's ribs, a lower daily caloric intake is called for.
2. While you're establishing the quantity of food to feed, you should weigh your cat every week. Since cats aren't dependable for sitting still on a scale, weigh yourself, then weigh yourself holding your cat. The difference in poundage is your cat's weight.
3. Once your cat is at optimal weight, keep the food quality high and adjust the amount fed daily to meet your pet's caloric needs.
4. Every month, after the diet has been established, weigh your cat to see that there isn't a weight loss or gain of more than 5 to 10 percent. If there is, increase or decrease the amount of daily food intake accordingly.

Getting-Acquainted Basic Breakfast

Try 1/4 to 1/3 cup of professional/alternative dry cat food (Iams; Feline Growth from Hill's; Pro Plan; Precise Feline Foundation). Available from pet stores and vets, these foods supply concentrated energy and nutrition.

If you wish, you may begin with any good-quality commercial dry food, but your new cat will have to consume a larger volume of food to meet its breakfast caloric requirement.

If your new pet refuses dry food and your veterinarian has found no existing dental problem, the cat's refusal could be the result of a prior gum or tooth condition. Or, it could simply be that the animal has never chewed dry food before. Since dry food can be a preventive for tartar buildup and potential dental problems, I feel it should be part of every cat's weekly diet. And the sooner you can get yours to enjoy it, the better.

How to Get Your Cat to Enjoy Dry Food

- Mix a few pieces of dry food in with the canned food.
- Increase the amount of dry as your cat gets accustomed to it, proportionately decreasing the amount of canned food. (Don't rush the process.)
- Once your cat will eat a completely dry food meal, feed only dry for three days in a row before offering canned food.

Breakfast Booster Treats

- Egg yolk or hard-boiled egg (can be added one to three times weekly)
- Cottage cheese (two tablespoons)
- Plain yogurt (two tablespoons)
- Bacon grease (1/4 teaspoon, one to three times weekly) added to the dry or canned food

Deluxe Dinner

Serve 3–4 oz. of canned professional/alternative cat food (Feline Growth (Hill's), Iams Cat Food, Precise, Pro Plan (Purina), Triumph,

to name a few). Refrigerate unused portion. (For optimal flavor retention, store in an airtight container instead of the can.) When reserving, don't forget to warm to room temperature by adding a little
hot water or broth, placing the bowl in a pan of hot water, or setting
the bowl in the microwave and reheating the contents until the
chill is gone. Test the food's temperature with your finger before
feeding. Never recook food and never serve leftover food cold!

It is not advisable to store canned food for more than two days.
To avoid waste, I'd suggest serving the remainder of a canned meal
the following morning for breakfast, and giving dry food for dinner.
If the food you're using comes in 15 oz. cans, and you find that you
still have leftovers, serve it for both meals the next day. The day
after that serve only dry food.

Deluxe Dinner Dividends

- Serve 1 teaspoon less of leftover canned food and replace with
  1–2 teaspoons cooked chicken, beef or fish. Limit to three
  times weekly, since professional foods are optimally balanced,
  and your goal is optimal nutrition.
- Mix 1/4–1/2 teaspoon of brewer's yeast or torula yeast into
  food. This provides extra B vitamins that can also help keep
  fleas away. It can be done daily.
- If you are not feeding a quality, nutritionally balanced food regularly, tasty cat vitamins will speed your stray's shape-up.
  (F-Biotic, Felovite, Dr Jane® Beezyme or Pro Balance are examples.)

For Best Results

- Feed no generic foods.
- Feed professional/alternative food from your veternarian or
  pet store.
- Give hair-ball medicine twice weekly.
- Comb and brush your pet daily. This helps prevent hair balls,
  which can cause stomach problems and undermine any nutrition regimen. It will also give you visible evidence of your cat's
  rapidly improving condition. Buy a comb with teeth spaced
  widely enough not to pull your cat's fur, yet narrow enough to

remove dead hair, flaky skin and possible parasite eggs. If mats won't comb out, snip with blunt children's scissors. Use a soft-bristle brush that will stimulate your pet's oil glands. Brush from tail to neck, neck to tail, then back again.

Your cat might not be able to say how much it appreciates New-Life nutrition, but it will surely show it. (A healthy coat speaks for itself.) Within two weeks the benefits will be obvious; within four weeks they will be irrefutable.

New-Life for Your Beloved Older Cat

Just because a cat can't stay young doesn't mean it can't stay healthy.

Once upon a time, early in my career, I had the good fortune to adopt a cat named Cinderella. She was a beautiful, silvery, deep gray, domestic shorthair of magically mixed breed, a combination of kittenish mischief and feline formidability. According to her medical file, she was six years old with no physical problems and her appearance and behavior gave me no reason to doubt it.

But her file was only partially correct. Cinderella was sixteen, not six. The record's inaccuracy was due to a typo; Cinderella's youthfulness was due to her owner's sixteen years of unswerving, enlightened, nutritional care.

What I learned from this fairy-godmother owner was what I had always believed; growing old doesn't have to mean looking, or feeling, old. Recognizing that a cat's nutritional needs vary with age—as well as with breed, physical condition, household environment, even changes in weather—is necessary for keeping your pet in optimal condition.

How Old Is Old? A cat that celebrates his tenth birthday, and any thereafter, by bounding effortlessly on the counter for a preview of dinner is not one that you might deem old; but, visible or not, aging changes have begun. Dietary modifications must be considered if you want your pet to continue celebrating birthdays in equivalent good health.

Not all cats age at the same rate or in the same fashion, but with increasing years all will experience the effects of aging. The aging process can not be stopped, but it can be slowed with good preventive nutrition.

Familiarizing yourself with changes and resulting problems that can occur with aging will help you decide what food adjustments are best for your individual cat.

As Your Cat Ages

Changes	Possible Problems
Decreased thyroid function and basal metabolism	Obesity, due to lower energy needs and slowing down of all body functions
Decreased sense of smell, diminished intake of nutrients	Appetite loss, weight loss, not enough vital nutrients
Decreased sensitivity to thirst	Dehydration, kidney disease
Decreased ability to regulate body temperature for warmth or cooling	Increased susceptibility to illness, nervousness, irritability
Increased thyroid function and basal metabolism (hyperthyroidism)	Thin, nervous, weak, heart problem
Decreased immune system effectiveness	Increased susceptibility to illness
Decreased liver function	Increased susceptibility to toxins; diminished drug tolerance and ability to properly digest and utilize necessary fats and other nutrients; digestive problems
Decreased pancreas function	Impaired food digestion and assimilation, gastrointestinal upsets, increased chances of diabetes mellitus

Changes	Possible Problems
Tooth and gum degeneration	Insufficient food intake because of impaired chewing ability, vomiting, bad breath, bacterial infections throughout the body
Decreased salivary secretion	Insufficient nutrient intake, vomiting, constipation
Decreased restful sleep	Unexplained irritability and other behavioral quirks
Decreased visual and hearing acuity	Irritability; increased susceptibility to environmental hazards; increased stress, vomiting and loss of equilibrium due to inner-ear degeneration
Decreased intestinal absorption	Insufficient intake of all nutrients; calcium deficiency causing osteoporosis (brittle bones), gas, diarrhea, constipation, odorous stools, weight loss
Decreased colon motility	Constipation
Decreased skin elasticity; drying, thinning, and coarsening of coat; excessive or decreased production of oil glands	Increased susceptibility to skin diseases
Decreased kidney (renal) function	Generalized kidney disease, gastric ulcers, excessive drinking and urination, incontinence

Changes	Possible Problems
Muscular-skeletal degeneration	Flaccid abdominal and other visible muscles as well as cardiac (heart) muscles, arthritis, back stiffness, poor coordination of limbs
Decreased cardiovascular function	Heart disease, arteriosclerosis, easily fatigued
Decreased respiratory function	Chronic bronchitis, tumors in respiratory system, asthma, fatigue
Decreased neurological function	Slow response to stimuli, memory loss, impaired sensory reactions (sight, sound, smell, taste)

New Ways to Feed and Nurture an Older Cat
(also see my 30-days regimen for senior cats)

- Feed smaller, easily digestible, quality, balanced, high-BV-protein meals more frequently, three or four times daily. This eases the stress on internal organs, keeps the immune system strong and keeps your pet's energy level from falling.
- Avoid all generic foods.
- Avoid feeding meals with imbalanced essential fatty acids or those with incorrect or insufficient nutrients to utilize fat. This can prevent flaking, dry skin and a wide variety of coat and skin problems. Supplements such as Dr. Jane® Essential Gold, Pet Tabs F.A., or any others that contain Vitamin E and balanced fatty acids can help.
  NOTE: Always read the supplement label to make sure that all necessary fatty acids are included.
- Count calories and make those calories count—a fat cat is not going to be a fit cat.
- Don't feed your cat baby food. The calcium/phosphorus ratio is wrong for felines and can worsen many health problems.

- Brush your older pet daily and give hair-ball medication two or three times a week.
- Make sure your cat has fresh water every day—and that your cat drinks it.
- Dehydration is not uncommon in older cats because of their decreased thirst sensitivity. If you find that your cat isn't drinking, add a bit of water (or warm broth, clam juice or tomato juice) to your cat's meals.
- As cats grow older, their calcium needs increase. A deficiency can cause brittle bones (osteoporosis). Adding sardines to your pet's diet (provided the cat doesn't have FLUTD), is a way to provide extra calcium that even finicky eaters appreciate. Mash the sardines before adding to your pet's food, and remember that the addition shouldn't be more than 25 percent of the meal. Cottage cheese is another easy-to-enjoy calcium booster for older cats.
- Brewer's yeast or torula yeast with bran (which contains the B complex vitamins and fiber) and vitamin C (200–300 mg), are excellent stress fighters and constipation preventives. I recommend supplementing an older cat's diet with both daily. (If using the ester powdered form of vitamin C, 1/8 teaspoon is approximately 500 mg.) Antioxidants definitely help slow aging; you can select a formula that has a combination of antioxidants such as C, E, or beta-carotene (Dr. Jane® Feline Formula One with taurine, essential oils and antioxidants).
- Raw garlic adds potassium and boosts the immune system. Add 1/8–1/4 teaspoon to your senior's food.
- If your pet is not eating a quality professional/alternative food, I'd recommend giving a multiple vitamin-mineral supplement with amino acids and fatty acids such as Pro Balance, F-Biotic or Dr. Jane® Beezyme daily. *CAUTION*: If your cat has any existing medical problems, check with your vet before making any dietary additions or changes.
- Enzymes will help digest the needed nutrients from food. If you are not adding Dr. Jane® Beezyme (which contains vegetable enzyme) then Prozyme or Florazyme is a must. It can increase nutrient uptake by 25–30% and will not alter your cat food balance.
- A little extra attention goes a long way in keeping a cat youthful, especially if you give that attention in the form of exercise

play. The exercise should not, of course, be excessive or exhausting. My twelve-year-old Rex, Jeddy, loved stalking and swatting bubbles and pursuing any toy that rolls downstairs. And you'll be surprised at how short walks can work energizing wonders.

- Because older cats are often candidates for respiratory problems, keeping a humidifier in your home during the winter months is advisable.
- Don't forget about sunlight! It plays an important part in the well-being of cats of all ages and is particularly important for older cats. Sunlight provides vitamin D, which is vital for bone growth and maintenance as well as effective metabolization of calcium. If you have an indoor cat, be aware that ordinary glass windows do not let in the essential ultraviolet rays. There are, however, special types of plastic windows that do. Your local hardware store should be able to tell you about them. You can also buy a special "full spectrum" artificial light that provides proper light for cats of all ages and is particularly important for older ones.

Super Supper Picker-Upper
for Senior Cats

A special once-or-twice-a-week treat created for pampering your pet.

Super Supper Picker-Upper

2–3 ounces cooked chicken (no skin) or boneless fish (haddock, sole, flounder)	1 eggshell, cooked and finely ground, or 1 pulverized 50 mg calcium tablet
1/8 teaspoon canned pumpkin	1/8 teaspoon wheat germ oil
1/8 teaspoon brewer's yeast or torula yeast	1 tablespoon cottage cheese
	1 tablespoon cooked oatmeal

Mix all ingredients well. If your cat prefers a more moist consistency, add 1–2 tablespoons of water or warm broth. (Approximately 180 calories)

Q&A

My cat Horatio is probably fourteen years old. I have been feeding him just as I always did from the day I got him at age two. I guess it happened overnight, or I hadn't been paying attention, but he looks thin and "rough." He drinks water all day (guess I didn't notice because he drinks from the faucet) and seems weak. It's hard to tell because he sleeps most of the time. What type of dietary regimen do you recommend?

Older cats do have different needs than younger ones (see page 148: New Life for Your Beloved Older Cat). While a healthy cat may be able to cope with a deficient diet, an older cat simply can't and will begin to show symptoms of dietary distress quickly. I recommend that all owners re-evaluate their senior cats' diets to adjust for their life requirements (see page 151 on geriatric diet).

While Hills, Purina and other food manufacturers have formulated senior feline diets, I don't feel that they have addressed many of the special senior nutritional requirements. While these diets tend to contain fewer calories, which I agree with, I am not enthusiastic about their high fiber. I currently recommend that unless your senior cat (over 10 years of age) is overweight, that you feed it a high-quality alternative professional food, adding the supplements I have recommended in this book.

Your cat doesn't sound like it's a candidate for a simple diet change. He needs to visit the family veterinarian *now*. Horatio has to be examined and tested for kidney disease, diabetes mellitus and other aging diseases. His diet will depend upon the medical findings. If he has kidney disease, he will begin a specially formulated food. Potassium, B vitamins and vegetable enzymes would be very helpful, but discuss any dietary changes with your veterinarian.

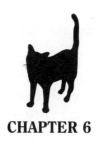

CHAPTER 6

. . . .

Special Needs
of Special Breeds

. . . .

The following food and supplement recommendations are not intended to be prescriptive. Before making changes in your cat's diet, consult your veterinarian to be sure that your pet has no special physical problems, or is taking no medication that might cause contraindicate alterations in the animal's present diet.

Abyssinian

Shorthaired, firm and muscular, this lithe and fast-moving cat with the exotic look of an ancient Egyptian animal god is known for its sleek, shiny coat and unbounded playfulness. Its diet must contain ample protein and balanced fatty acids to meet high-energy requirements and maintain a coat in good condition. They can usually "free feed"; because they are so active, they burn off extra calories—couch potatoes they are not.

Many Abyssinians are prone to gingivitis, so I recommend feeding a quality professional/alternative dry food at least three to five times a week to help prevent tartar buildup and keep gums healthy. Also give 100–200 mg of vitamin C everyday.

155

If you are using supermarket-label food, add a well-rounded supplement with vitamins, minerals, amino acids and fats (see pages 86-99). Hot milk before bed may help calm him. Brewer's or turula yeast given daily will supply the B vitamins that could take the "edge" off this active cat. Hops can be added, especially when the cat is particularly active.

American Shorthair

The classic-touch, sturdy alley cat is big in size and has an appetite to match. Optimally, these cats should be rounded and robust, firm and not flabby. Unfortunately, obesity is all too common in the breed.

To prevent your American Shorthair from becoming a flabby tabby, once a month gently pinch his sides. You should always be able to feel the cat's ribs without difficulty. If you can't, a calorie cutback is in order. Avoid feeding this lusty feline any foods with a high cereal content, don't leave meals down all day and skip the bedtime snacks.

Exercise is the key to fitness. Provide 5–10 minutes of exercise three times a day if you can.

American Curl

A rounded, robust, but relatively small cat, with curly hair in the ears, these cats need a well-balanced diet with a brewer's yeast and garlic supplement that will enhance their beautiful coats.

American Wirehair

Because of the breed's lightly curled, springy coat, it's important that this cat's hairs grow evenly—unless, of course, you don't mind living with an animal that will look like a used Brillo pad on paws. Since the coat is the first area to show nutritional deficiencies, a balanced diet is essential. Avoid feeding table scraps and treats that could interfere with the Wirehair's intake of quality protein and fat. Add a vegetable enzyme or Dr. Jane® Beezyme for insurance.

Balinese and Javanese

Longhaired and active, these elegant and inquisitive felines require frequent brushing. They're also high-spirited (occasionally too high) and use their B vitamins faster than you can name them. A simple remedy is to add 1/8–1/4 teaspoon of brewer's yeast or torula yeast to their meals.

To help prevent dull, cottonlike coats (a frequent problem), as well as dry, flaking skin, these cats should receive a balanced, fatty-acid supplement with zinc once a day or Dr. Jane® Feline Formula One. Hair-ball medication should be given two to three times weekly, between meals.

Birman

This large, pensive, silky-haired cat with white-gloved paws loves company; to look and feel its best when socializing, it should be kept in proper condition.

Essential fatty acids are a must, along with sufficient vitamin E in the diet to utilize them. If you're not providing a high-protein, high-fat alternative food, supplement meals with 1/4 teaspoon bacon grease or, preferably, a balanced store-bought fatty-acid formula with zinc or Dr. Jane® Feline Formula One. I'd also recommend adding bee pollen. The bee pollen will supply the additional micronutrients these gentle giants need.

A diet that promotes steady, firm growth from kittenhood will keep your Birman muscular, instead of fat, and sleek for life. Don't forget hair-ball medicine.

Bombay

Of medium size, this muscular extrovert's most outstanding feature is its soft, glossy coat. If you rub it with a chamois cloth it will glow. Complete and balanced foods, with high-BV protein, all the essential fatty acids, and zinc, are daily diet necessities. But watch out! The Bombay enjoys meals and has a tendency to overeat. Feed him quality, not quantity.

If you are using supermarket-label food, add a well-rounded supplement with vitamins, minerals, amino acids, fats (see pages 86 and 87) or supplement with plants or herbs, such as bee pollen, Dr. Jane® Beezyme, algae, or parsley, rather than synthetic vitamins and minerals.

Bengal

This wild-looking cat needs an alternative food for sure. The plush fur really looks its best when brewer's or torula yeast is added to the diet.

These cats can put on weight, so make sure that you exercise them, and don't give them the snacks they so often desire.

British Shorthair

Large and placid with an impressive thick coat, a British Short-hair's favorite pastimes are sleeping and eating, with play being least important. Since this breed's relatively inactive lifestyle is conducive to obesity and FLUTD, maximum nutrition must be provided in minimum quantity.

Feed only twice daily. Do not leave food out for all-day nibbling.

Avoid feeding red fish and foods high in magnesium. (See chapter 4 for low-magnesium foods.) Meat protein is a must to keep the urine slightly acidic.

Always keep fresh water available.

If you're not providing a quality professional/alternative diet, I'd suggest giving a balanced supplement once a day.

Brewer's yeast or torula yeast will keep that plush coat glamourous!

Burmese

An active show-off with a stunning sable-brown coat that any feline would envy, the Burmese is a combination stand-up (and roll-over) comic and Olympic athlete.

The breed is prone to ocular discharge, so supplementing the diet with vitamin C, 100–200 mg daily, or an antioxidant formula, is recommended. I've found this helpful in averting potential eye problems and clearing up those that already exist.

For continued coat beauty, feed a professional/alternative high-quality food plus a supplement that enhances the beautiful coat and protects from allergies. Torula yeast and garlic or brewer's yeast is the perfect, healthy treat.

Chartreux

A large, gentle powerhouse of a cat, the Chartreux is a smiler, a jumper, a hunter and great for multi-pet households. Its thick bluish coat is plush and should glisten. Though capable of numerous activities, it has a tendency to be lazy and often enjoys entire afternoons just sunbathing.

His coat should be shiny, not at all dull. If your cat isn't being fed a professional/alternative food, give him a well-rounded balanced supplement daily (see pages 86 and 87).

Do not overfeed. Once a month, gently pinch your pet's side to be sure you can still feel his ribs. A Chartreux can easily become very chubby. Exercise is a must.

Feed low-magnesium foods. The incidence of FLUTD is frequent. Add 1–2 tablespoons of tomato juice to moist food three to five times weekly and supplement the diet with 200 mg of ester-powdered vitamin C daily.

Colorpoint Shorthair

Essentially, and for all nutritional purposes, this breed is Siamese with color variations. (See Siamese.)

Cornish Rex

This is a curvy cat, structured somewhat like a small greyhound, whose wavy, plush, rippled coat makes it an eye-catching pet. It is not necessarily less allergenic than other cats. Active and energetic, the Cornish Rex is a rugged cat, despite its delicate frame. It still sheds, so hair-ball medication should be given once a week.

These cats have a high metabolism (their normal body temperature is slightly above that of other breeds) and huge appetites. Do not allow free feeding! As energetic as the Cornish Rex is, it can easily overeat and become a blimp. It needs food with quality protein and usable fat for meeting its energy needs including keeping warm. This breed is not meant for cold climates or cold weather. I recommend keeping a T-shirt on a Rex from October to May. If he has problems with the cold, add garlic to the diet every day.

The tail area has a tendency to become oily if the diet is insufficient in usable fat, vitamin E, and zinc. Shampoo wipes are handy to clean the tail once in a while. Brush the coat with a soft brush, but do it gently.

If you're not feeding your Rex a professional/alternative food, I would suggest adding a well-rounded supplement with vitamins, minerals, amino acids and fats (see page 87).

Cymric

The long and short of this cat are its hair and its front legs. It has no tail to speak of—and shouldn't—since it is the longhaired version of the distinctly tailless Manx breed, from which it descended. The Cymric is also called the Long-Haired Manx.

Because of the Cymric's unusual body symmetry with its raised muscular hindquarters and short front legs, a well-known brand professional/alternative food is a must. Proper calcium and mineral balance is essential. Cottage or ricotta cheese three times weekly is a simple and effective way to ensure calcium.

All-meat diets are a definite no! The high phosphorus/calcium ratio can be detrimental.

Quality, high-BV protein and balanced fatty acids are necessary for adequate muscle growth and for keeping this cat's double coat shining. If you're not feeding a professional/alternative food regularly, add a well-rounded supplement with vitamins, minerals, amino acids and fats (see page 87).

Brush and comb your Cymric two or three times a week. Give hair-ball medicine twice weekly between meals.

Devon Rex

A slightly larger, fuzzier, longer-haired but more delicate version of the Cornish Rex. The same high-fat, quality protein, protective warmth and supplement needs apply.

Egyptian Mau

Still a rare breed, this muscular and stealthy predator is a hardy, medium-sized shorthair with a slick, spotted, leopardlike coat. Its hind legs are longer than the front, so balanced calcium is essential. Its nutritional needs are basic and met easily with a well-balanced feline diet. Brewer's or torula yeast is great for its coat.

Exercise will help keep your cat in good muscular condition.

Exotic Shorthair

If you can imagine a sort of low-maintenance, laid-back, short-haired Persian, you've a pretty good idea of an Exotic Shorthair. This cat is easier to groom than a Persian, but sufficiently balanced fatty acids and a high-BV-protein diet are nonetheless essential for the health of its lush fur coat. Torula yeast is an excellent supplement for these FLUTD-prone cats. Hair-ball remedies twice weekly are a must.

Similar to Persians, Exotic Shorthairs are prone to eye discharge and infections. It's therefore advisable to supply them with 200 mg of extra vitamin C daily or an antioxidant formula.

Havana Brown

This is a hardy, adaptable cat who is full of fun and plays very well with others, but has a tendency to want its owner's undivided attention. It has many character and physical traits of a Siamese.

The Havana's shorthair coat requires minimal grooming (once a week is fine), but to keep it lustrous, this cat should be given a balanced fatty-acid supplement with vitamins and minerals daily or an herbal supplement combined with a professional/alternative food (see pages 86 and 87).

Himalayan and Kashmir

Gentle, longhaired Persian types, these cats like to exercise and do well in roomy homes with other pets and children.

Himalayans and Kashmirs tend to have improperly developed tear ducts, causing discharge from the eyes. Because of their short noses, they're also more susceptible to respiratory disease. Vitamin C or an antioxidant formula should be given on a daily basis.

Conscientious daily coat combing is necessary to prevent tangled, cottony-looking fur. Vegetable enzymes or Dr. Jane® Beezyme are also essential. If your cat's coat is in poor condition, add torula yeast with the vegetable enzymes (but *not* with Dr. Jane® Beezyme). Torula yeast will keep the coat healthy. Hair-ball medication should be given two or three times weekly between meals.

Japanese Bobtail

Usually calico-patterned (red, black, and white), this unique feline—immortalized for centuries in Japanese artworks—is both reserved and playful. In fact, on a warm, summer day, a bob might even climb into a birdbath or shallow tub for a recreational splash. It's so inquisitive that it never seems to gain weight—so you can leave food down all day.

Easy to care for, your bob only really needs a balanced diet of alternative food and a daily antioxidant supplement.

Korat

If you're looking for an alert "guard cat," a well-bred Korat can't be beat. Properly aloof and often suspicious of strangers, this shorthair, with its extraordinary agility and fabulous silver-blue coat, is a regular James (or Jane) Bond on paws and is devoted to its owners.

Korats deserve nothing but the best in the way of nutrition, and they should get it—on schedule. Feed professional/alternative food regularly, with a daily vegetable enzyme and/or antioxidant formula.

If you are providing supermarket foods, I suggest giving your pet a balanced supplement with vitamin, minerals, fat and amino acids (see pages 86 and 87).

Maine Coon

At first glance, you might think it's a dog in drag, and with good reason. This is a large cat. At ten months, my nephew's Maine Coon, George, was nineteen pounds of muscular machismo and had taken a lion's share of awards at the Empire Cat Show.

My advice for keeping a Maine Coon in keen shape is to feed it high-BV-protein nutritionally balanced meals three to four times daily (no free feeding). If you are using supermarket-label food, add a well-rounded supplement with vitamins, minerals, amino acids and fats (see pages 86 and 87). This will supply correctly proportioned amounts of energy, keeping the cat muscular and active. You do not want a fat Maine Coon, believe me—obesity problems aside, you could get a hernia just carrying him to the vet!

As big as Maine Coons are, they are gentle, loving, adaptable to all sorts of household situations and climates, and they make terrific pets. A regular, weekly combing should be enough to keep their coats tangle-free, but you may want to add brewer's or torula yeast for that "extra" hair conditioning, and don't forget hair-ball medicine!

Malayan

A purebred Malayan is a bit more assertive than a Burmese, but its nutritional needs are the same. (See Burmese.)

Manx

Of medium size, this tailless, wily cat is deceptively powerful. Its awkward gait and build are genetic, not caused by a nutritional deficiency.

The Manx's thick, double coat needs regular brushing and a good fatty-acid supplement with zinc. The calcium phosphorous ratio must not be compromised by the addition of a supplement to a professional/alternative food. If you are feeding an alternative food, add Dr. Jane® Beezyme or bee pollen, but if you are feeding a super-market-label food, add a well-rounded supplement with vitamins, minerals, amino acids and fats (see pages 86 and 87).

Personality-wise, a Manx is a one-person pet, perfect for single owners. They love to play and exercise, which will keep their weight down.

Norwegian Forest Cat

If cats could ski, the Norwegian Forest Cat would be the first on the slopes, and undoubtedly—because it thrives on companionship—a hit at the ski lodge.

Its thick, double coat is not only beautiful, but also water-resistant and will stay tangle free. I'd recommend daily combing to slough off dead hair and cells, which will help prevent hair balls as well as stimulate the oil glands that keep the coat water-resistant. Needless to say, hair-ball medicine two times weekly is a must!

Make sure this cat is eating a professional/alternative diet of high-BV protein. Vegetable enzymes will ensure that all essential hair nutrients get delivered. Brewer's or torula yeast will certainly keep the coat healthy. They love to nibble on grass, so grow some wheat grass.

Ocicat

This large, imposing, sleek shorthair has the look of a feral feline, but is in every sense of the word a pussycat—sweet, bright and gentle.

This is essentially a very healthy cat and is easily kept that way by avoiding food with too much cereal filler and sticking to a high-BV-protein diet. Its beautiful marked coat will glow with the addition of a fatty-acid supplement.

Ocicats are, however, prone to nervousness. Supplementing their diet with B complex vitamins—1/8–1/4 teaspoon brewer's or torula yeast mixed with food daily—calms their nerves; however some swear by hot milk or crushed hops added to their food.

Oriental Shorthair

Distinctively elegant, agile, and loving, the Oriental Shorthair is a thinner, more muscular, almost-identical twin to the Siamese. Not surprisingly, the two breeds have the same nutritional needs. These are listed in detail under "Siamese."

Persian

The Persian is the quintessential, luxuriously longhaired, and usually royally pampered cat. Unfortunately, many of the Persians I've seen have been pampered to death by indulgent, nutritionally uneducated owners.

The major errors, I've found, are feeding all-meat diets, baby food, overfeeding with table scraps and treats, and leaving food down for all-day nibbling. These are definite—and dangerous no-nos!

Persians are not particularly active cats and are prone to obesity and FLUTD; proper diet is, therefore, a necessity. Calorie intake should be controlled. Feed only low-magnesium foods. You may want to leave food down all day for those predisposed to FLUTD.

Ocular discharge is common in this breed, so you should clean a Persian's eyes once or twice daily with a piece of damp, sterile cotton. To prevent eye infections, a strong immune system must be present to provide ample antibodies. A daily antioxidant plus bee pollen should be given. If you are using supermarket-label food, add a well-rounded supplement with vitamins, minerals, amino acids and fats (see pages 86 and 87). A specific hair supplement containing the vitamins B, zinc, and fatty acids can make that marvelous coat look its very best.

With Persians, grooming can not be ignored and should be done daily. Remember, when brushing, brush backwards to distribute oils evenly. Administer hair-ball medication between meals two or three times weekly. Vegetable enzyme will ensure delivery of essential hair and coat nutrients, and help break apart hair balls.

Ragdoll

Related to the Persian, this exceptionally large, longhaired cat is happiest when not in motion. To call it mellow is an understatement; to arouse its interest in anything other than food or sleep is an achievement. Despite its size, it's the perfect pet for small apartments.

Nutritionally, the Ragdoll's needs are the same as a Persian's, but you'll find that it requires considerably less grooming because its coat doesn't mat as easily. Hair-ball medication should be given between meals two or three times weekly.

Russian Blue

A svelte, aloof shorthair, this cat sports a lush thick, double coat that often conceals excess pounds if feeding isn't carefully supervised. The Russian Blue tends to lounge more than leap, making it an easy target for obesity and FLUTD.

Since its coat is its major feature, brushing is a must. You don't want to dull this cat's exquisite fur. Brush it backwards then forwards daily. This will stimulate oil glands, remove dead hair, and keep the coat shiny without flattening it. Give hair-ball medication between meals once or twice a week. A hair supplement with fatty acids, B vitamins and zinc is advisable.

If you're not providing a professional/alternative diet regularly, give a balanced supplement daily, but a professional/alternative food is really what it should have.

Though this breed is usually gentle, I've seen quite a few unruly Russian Blues. If yours is one, I'd suggest supplementing its meals with a balanced 25–50 mg B vitamin supplement and mixing 1–2 tablespoons of chamomile tea in moist food daily. Start with 1 teaspoon and gradually increase the amount.

Scottish Fold

Known for its folded-down ears and soulful eyes, this well-behaved and amiable cat is surprisingly hardy. Feeding yours a good balanced diet of high-BV protein and fat can keep it that way.

I would suggest, however, that since the Scottish Fold is particularly susceptible to ear mites, you should supplement its daily diet with garlic (1/8 teaspoon) and brewer's or torula yeast. If ear mites are present, you'll need special medication from the veterinarian to kill them. In any event, cleaning your cat's ears once a week with a cotton swab dampened in a mild hydrogen peroxide solution is a must for averting serious potential problems.

Exercise will help keep their compact, firm, muscular bodies healthy.

Siamese

The Siamese is unquestionably the cat most likely to want things its own way—and usually gets it. Incredibly intelligent, ingenious, agile and active, this dauntless, ultrasleek and slender feline has a mind of its own, and you never know what it will think of next.

To meet its high-energy needs and still retain its long, lean beauty (a show Siamese must have absolutely minimum fat and muscle over its rib cage), this cat requires high-BV protein and balanced fatty acids daily. Commercial foods with a high cereal or carbohydrate content should be avoided, as should raw-meat diets (these can cause muscle flaccidity and hair loss). On the other hand, nondigestible carbohydrates (fiber), such as beet pulp or grated carrots, should be included in your Siamese's diet. These will cleanse intestine walls, preventing bowel problems, and keep it from getting fat. If there is a fiber insufficiency, you'll soon find your genius rectifying it by chewing socks, sweatshirts, towels and so on. Growing kitty greens could save you lots of socks.

For a very active Siamese, a little nutritional calming can be obtained by supplementing the diet with a balanced Vitamin B complex or 1/8–1/4 teaspoon brewer's yeast or torula yeast daily. I give mine chamomile tea (1/4 teaspoon in its food); this seems to help him digest while keeping him calm. I add hops to his evening meal, which allows everyone to sleep during the night.

Siamese love to fetch, so make 10–20 aluminum balls and throw them every night. Exercise is a must for these cats.

Singapura
Small and shorthaired, this breed is very similar to the Abyssinian (see above). This breed may also require chamomile and/or hops.

Snowshoe
This breed is not quite as large as a Maine Coon (see above), but it has the same basic temperament, sociability, fortitude and nutritional needs.

Somali
An active and often acrobatic longhair whose theme song is "Don't Fence Me In," this fun-loving feline likes room to play.

A Somali needs high-BV protein and quality fat. If you're not feeding yours a professional/alternative food, give him a balanced supplement with vitamins, minerals and fatty acids, as well as an egg yolk (no uncooked whites) twice weekly.

Many Somalis have a tendency to be hyper as well as active, usually in the evening when you're ready for sleep. If yours is a late night partier, a vitamin B complex or 1/8–1/4 teaspoon brewer's yeast is a smart daily meal supplement, along with a nightcap of room-temperature chamomile tea, or lactose-free warm milk and honey. Ground or chopped hops added to the evening meal may also help keep peace in the family.

Sphinx

A fabulous, fragile feline, virtually hairless, the Sphinx needs special care and clothing (it should wear a sweater or T-shirt at all times, except in the tropics) and requires a truly dedicated owner who will not only protect it from the cold but also provide it with absolutely optimal nutrition. Garlic will help keep its immune system healthy throughout the winter months. Because of this cat's extra-high metabolism, obesity isn't a problem, but supplying adequate nutrition is.

A professional/alternative high-quality meat diet, plus antioxidants and bee pollen are a must. A raw egg yolk (no uncooked whites) can be added to meals two or three times a week.

Shampoo wipes are useful to clean the accumulated saliva, which can make the coat sticky.

Tiffany

This is the longhaired version of a Burmese. Its nutritional needs are the same, though the Tiffany requires more grooming and should get hair-ball medication between meals once or twice a week. Vegetable enzyme or Dr. Jane® Beezyme will ensure a good-looking coat.

Tonkinese

A delightful, mischievous, quality combination of Siamese and Burmese, the Tonkinese has basically the same nutritional and supplemental needs as both the Siamese and the Burmese, but tends to eat more than either. Obesity can cause your Tonkinese serious problems, so be careful not to overfeed. No free feeding.

Also keep in mind that a Tonkinese, similar to a Siamese, has a definite intestine-cleansing need for fiber. If there are fiber insufficiencies in your pet's diet, you're likely to find that there will be insufficiencies in your sweaters, socks, and towels as well. Grow wheat grass so your cat can get enough healthy fiber. These cats can have ocular discharge, so an antioxidant formula or vitamin C is needed. Catnip tea may help keep his chatter to a minimum.

Turkish Angora

This tall feline is a sociable, trainable, longhaired beauty who enjoys hunting, playing and even taking a splash in the tub now and then.

High-BV protein and fat are diet essentials, as is a good daily hair supplement. Vegetable enzyme or Dr. Jane® Beezyme will ensure a good coat and help break down hair balls as they form. In any event, give hair-ball medicine two or three times a week between meals.

Avoid giving your cat foods with dyes in them. These can discolor your cat's mane.

Q&A

Siamese and Their Bizarre Taste for Wool, Cotton, and Other Nonedibles

I have had Siamese cats all my life, and they ALL love to carry and sometimes eat my socks, cotton balls, dish towels and sweatshirts. I woke up one night with a hole in my sweatshirt the size of a quarter, and my Siamese started on a second. Why do they do this?

We are aware of this idiosyncracy, but are not sure exactly what causes it, or how to stop it. I suggest feeding more than three meals daily, so that hunger is not a reason. High-fiber food may help if it's fiber your cat needs. Growing kitty greens is an absolute must, as is feeding it a professional/alternative food with a vegetable enzyme to ensure the most complete digestion of nutrients possible.

Try to buy different textures of toys. A child's small stuffed animal is also a possible solution. Playing fetch with small, foam golf balls seems to keep some Siamese away from the laundry.

Hairless Ears Fears

Three months ago, I was given a dark, reddish brown, altered male cat that I was told was a purebred American Shorthair with no health problems. He's playful, loves to climb on my shoulder, has a fine, shiny coat and looks physically fit—except he has no hair on his ears. Have you any idea what could be causing this?

My guess is genetics. If your pet is indeed a purebred American Shorthair, it's probably a Havana Brown, a breed with naturally hairless ears.

Do Nonallergic Cats Really Exist?

I am allergic to cats and love them so much. My friends tell me the Sphinx is a "nonallergic" cat. Are they correct?

I am afraid there is no such animal. People are allergic to different components of the cat—saliva, dander and hair. While the Sphinx doesn't have hair, it still has dander and still produces saliva. If you are NOT allergic to dander, but are allergic to hair, then a Sphinx is your solution.

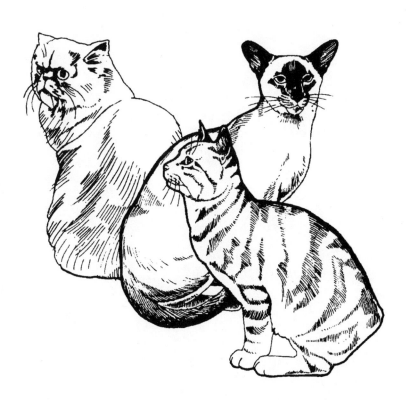

Part Three

· ·

Getting Better All the Time

· ·

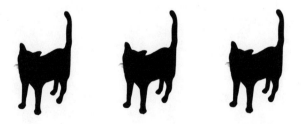

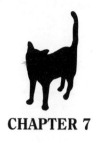

CHAPTER 7

....

Getting Physical

....

The Home Health Checkup

Giving your cat a simple monthly examination can prevent potential problems for years.

We all have a tendency to take our pets for granted, but you're making a big mistake if you do so. Cat owners, in particular, share the erroneous belief that their four-footed companions know what's best for them and rarely think about their pet's diet or health until the animal becomes visibly ill.

The truth is, smart as cats are, you're smarter. With minimal effort—essentially a once-a-month home examination and yearly veterinarian exam, you can avert a variety of problems and unnecessary trips to the vet, and keep your cat as fit as it ought to be for life.

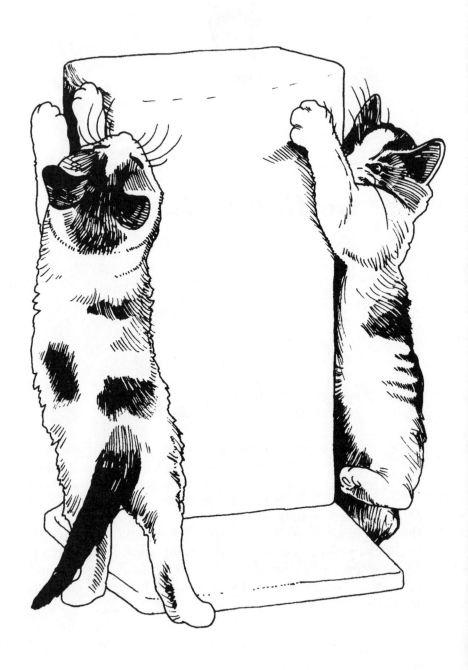

The Quick Cat Scan

	Yes	No
1. Have you noticed any recent changes in your cat's attitude or behavior, such as listlessness, restlessness, loss of appetite, aggression?	☐	☐
2. Does your cat's coat look dull or feel dry, brittle, or greasy?	☐	☐
3. Are his whiskers short or broken?	☐	☐
4. Using your hand, brush your cat's hair backwards from tail to head. His skin should be a normal grayish white. Is the skin a healthy color, or is it red and irritated? Is the tail area greasy with sparse hair?	☐	☐
5. Also look carefully for fleas or any little black flecks (the excrement of fleas) on skin. Do you see any?	☐	☐
6. Does the neck, back or base of the tail show any lesions?	☐	☐
7. Smell your hand after running it through your cat's fur. Your fingers should not have an unpleasant, fishy, rancid odor.	☐	☐
8. Are you able to feel good muscle tone around the sternum (breastbone)? It should not be soft or flaccid.	☐	☐
9. Do you feel a firm muscle mass when you run your hand down your cat's spine and over the rib cage? There should not be more than a pinch of fat	☐	☐
10. Open your cat's mouth and smell his breath. It should smell clean and not have an offensive odor. Does it smell clean?	☐	☐
11. Look at the gums. They should be pink, not pale or white, nor should they be swollen, bright red, or bleeding.	☐	☐

(continued)

	Yes	No
12. Check the teeth. Do they look white and healthy? They should be free of tartar and not loose.	☐	☐
13. Examine your cat's eyes. Are they clear of film and free of mucous discharge? Is there any crusting around them?	☐	☐
14. Feel the inner side of your cat's thighs. Are there any roundish bumps or swellings? These could indicate enlarged lymph nodes and usually the presence of worms.	☐	☐
15. Is your pet's stomach unusually distended?	☐	☐
16. Look at the paw pads. Are they smooth without dry, cracking lines?	☐	☐

Problems

What if your physical exam uncovers problems?

Besides doing the Quick Cat Scan, you should recognize your cat's daily habits and activities, which include behavior, bathroom habits (and I don't mean being neat about the litter box), vomiting, diarrhea and/or appetite. If you detect a problem, the following may help if it is a nutritional problem or, if it would respond to a nutritional change.

All you have to do is look up the problem in the following pages, they are listed according to main subject area, and see if any of the listed diet problems are similar to yours. Once you've identified that a potential health problem MAY be caused by diet, look up the solution in the various chapters of the book. Please keep in mind that if your cat is truly sick—go to your veterinarian. You may use the PROBLEM/ SOLUTION charts another time, or after your family veterinarian has seen your cat. I wish that all feline maladies were nutritionally induced, or responded to nutritional therapy, but they don't. So remember when I name a problem, vomiting for example, I DID NOT include causes, which could be medical in nature; such as a foreign body, liver or kidney disease, cancer, poison, etc.

Problems/Solutions

Attitude (Listlessness and Apathy)

POSSIBLE DIET PROBLEM	FINDING HELP
Increasing malnutrition due to poor quality cat food nutrient, inadequacy of home-cooked meals, or not feeding enough food	See chapter 10 for a good restorative diet; See chapters 5 and 10 for recipes that are nutritionally balanced for your cat.
Need for additional supplement	See chapter 5 on vitamins, minerals.

Bad Breath

POSSIBLE DIET PROBLEM	FINDING HELP
Deficiency of B vitamins in diet	See chapter 2 for prevention of vitamin loss and vitamin B-rich foods.
Excess gas due to poor digestion of food	See chapter 4 for guide to cat food benefits and risks.
Worms or intestinal parasites	See chapter 11 for prevention and remedies.
Gum or tooth decay, sometimes caused by lack of dry food needed to keep teeth clean	See chapter 4 for cat foods that can help maintain dental health.

Crust Around Eyes or Mouth

POSSIBLE DIET PROBLEM	FINDING HELP
Zinc, biotin, and/or niacin deficiency	See chapter 2 for vitamin and mineral needs and best food supplements.

Diarrhea

POSSIBLE DIET PROBLEM	FINDING HELP
Overeating	See "Obesity" in chapter 11 for how to control your pet's eating.
Change in diet	See chapter 10 for how to ease your cat into a new food regimen.
Deficiency in vitamins A and E, other fat-soluble vitamins, and nutrients necessary for fat utilization	See chapter 2 for fat requirements and prevention of oxidation.
Rancid or decayed food	See chapter 4 for how—and how long—to keep cat food.
Large doses of vitamin C	See chapter 2 for needs and supplement cautions.
Insufficient natural bran or fiber in diet	See chapter 4 for well-balanced cat foods; See "Carbohydrates" in chapter 2 for how to supplement.
Raw egg white in diet, which can cause biotin deficiency	See chapter 3 for avoiding mealtime mistakes.
Too many carbohydrates in diet	See chapter 2 for nutrient needs and cautions.
Sensitivity to single food ingredient; all-meat or all-fish diet	See chapter 3 for common feeding mistakes and diet myths.

Dry, Flaking, or Oily Skin

POSSIBLE DIET PROBLEM	FINDING HELP
Wrong or insufficient protein, fats, or vitamins and minerals in diet	See chapter 2 for good and bad types of fats for cats, supplements, and foods to avoid.

Excessive Shedding (including scarce or brittle hair)

POSSIBLE DIET PROBLEM	FINDING HELP
Nutrient deficiency in food, most likely inadequate protein, fatty acids, and vitamins A, E, and B complex	See chapter 4 for balanced and complete diet. See chapter 2 for good natural sources that supply these nutrients.
All-meat syndrome, a raw-meat diet providing insufficient amounts of nutrients—and calcium, in particular—for adequate food metabolization	See chapter 3 for common feeding mistakes. See chapter 2 for nutrition requirements.
Worms and intestinal parasites	See chapter 11 for prevention and remedies.
All-fish diet, which can cause Vitamin E deficiency (steatitis)	See chapter 3 for feeding mistakes. See chapter 2 for nutrition requirements.

Lack of Appetite

POSSIBLE DIET PROBLEM	FINDING HELP
Diet change	See chapter 11 for how to ease cat into accepting new food.
Multi-nutrient deficiency in current food, particularly A, E, B vitamins and protein	See chapter 2 for nutrition requirements. See "Anorexia" in chapter 11 for foods to stimulate appetite.

Lack of Muscle Tone

POSSIBLE DIET PROBLEM	FINDING HELP
Calcium deficiency, particularly if muscle around sternum (breastbone) is flaccid	See chapter 7 for instructions on checking for muscle tone. See chapter 2 for preventing calcium deficiency.
Obesity; can't feel muscle mass—only fat—along cat's backbone and rib cage	See chapter 11 for dietary prevention and cure.
Undernourishment, particularly if you feel no muscle, only backbone	See chapter 11 for proper way to fatten a thin cat.
Inadequate utilization of nutrients or improper food; insufficient exercise, particularly in indoor cats	See chapter 6 and 9 for breed's special needs and characteristics.

Pale Mucous Membranes *(gums or eyelids)*

POSSIBLE DIET PROBLEM	FINDING HELP
Inadequate intake of protein, vitamins and necessary trace minerals; particularly iron, biotin and copper	See chapter 7 for how to examine your cat. See chapter 4 for foods that are nutritionally balanced. See chapter 2 on herbs.

Runny Eyes *(mucous discharge)*

POSSIBLE DIET PROBLEM	FINDING HELP
Insufficient vitamin A in diet, or addition of too many polyunsaturated fats (which can inhibit vitamin A usefulness); insufficient immune system	See chapter 3 for preventive measures. See chapter 2 for proper use of fats for cats.

Unhealthy Whiskers *(short, broken, thin)*

POSSIBLE DIET PROBLEM	FINDING HELP
Inadequate protein quality or intake, insufficient nutrients to utilize available protein; intestinal parasites	See chapter 2 for protein needs, why certain deficiencies occur, and how these can be prevented and rectified through diet. See chapters 5 and 6 for special age and breed needs.

Split Nails

POSSIBLE DIET PROBLEM	FINDING HELP
Insufficient intake of nutrients, such as vitamin A, vitamin E, iodine and protein	See chapter 2 for vitamin and mineral needs and avoiding deficiencies. See chapter 4 for evaluating pet foods.

Sores That Don't Heal

POSSIBLE DIET PROBLEM	FINDING HELP
Insufficient fat-soluble vitamins, protein, zinc, and vitamin C being metabolized in diet	See chapter 2 for how to make sure the nutrients your cat is getting are being used effectively.

Unhealthy Pads (cracked or broken)

POSSIBLE DIET PROBLEM	FINDING HELP
Not enough dietary fat or protein, or incorrect proportion of nutrients in food	See chapter 2 for proper nutrient requirements. See chapter 4 for evaluating pet foods.

Vomiting

POSSIBLE DIET PROBLEM	FINDING HELP
Feeding a food that is not nutritionally balanced for your cat's age or breed	See chapters 5 and 6 for your cat's special requirements.

POSSIBLE DIET PROBLEM	FINDING HELP
Cat is eating too quickly, perhaps because of the presence of other pets or being fed in a busy, stressful area	See chapter 3 for tips on how to avoid mealtime mistakes.
Food is too cold, causing gastrointestinal upset	See chapter 3 for suggestions on proper preparation
Food has been kept too long and spoiled; leftovers unfit for you are just as unfit for your cat	See chapter 4 for how to store cat food.
Hunger. This type of vomiting —usually of a yellow, frothy consistency—can occur when your cat's stomach is empty	See chapter 3 for how to adjust feeding schedules.
Vitamin B deficiency, commonly caused by poor-quality commercial foods, all red-meat diets, or stress	See chapter 4 for vitamin-deficient cat foods. See chapter 2 for other B-rich additions to your cat's diet.
Eating grass, most likely due to empty stomach—possibly from overeating, sometimes nutrient deficiency, or need for fiber	See chapter 3 for why cats eat plants.
Poor teeth and gums, causing gulping of food	See chapter 4 for how to prevent tooth decay. See chapter 5 for tips on feeding toothless cats.
Hair balls	See chapter 7 for prevention and remedies.
Worms and intestinal parasites	See chapter 11 for prevention and remedies.

POSSIBLE DIET PROBLEM	FINDING HELP
Too much vitamin C	See chapter 2 for needs and supplement cautions.
FLUTD (feline lower urinary tract syndrome) possibly caused by too much magnesium in diet or too much cereal	See chapter 11 for disease prevention, symptoms, and recommended diet.
Constipation (what won't go out one way, will come out another)	See "Carbohydrates" in chapter 2 for diet preventives and cures.

How to Give Supplements to Your Cats

*It's not fun, but when the job must be done,
you should know how to do it.*

Face it. Cats will never understand that when you give them supplements, you're only doing it for their own good. And even if they did understand, they still wouldn't enjoy the process. (Who would?) The giving and taking of supplements isn't a fun activity for either party involved, but it needn't be a major battle, either.

Pilling a Cat Painlessly

Coat the pill with butter, oil or chicken fat, keeping it out of your cat's sight but within reach of your right hand. Get comfortable on a couch in front of the TV, and put the cat on your lap with his back toward you and his eyes facing the nightly news. You can use the dining room table if that's easier.

Begin loving, petting and murmuring endearments, giving the cat time to forget any initial suspicion and time to relax. When you've got your pet purring, slyly stroke the sides of its face with the thumb and index finger of your left hand while surreptitiously picking up the pill with your right. Then, without flinching or breaking the mood, firmly force open the cat's mouth, tilting his head just slightly, and pop the pill in (as far back on the center of the tongue as possible). Quickly close the mouth, hold it (still murmuring softly), and gently stroke the cat's throat until it reflexively swallows. Keep petting and cooing for at least two more minutes, pretending that what has just happened was as much a surprise to you as it was for your cat.

Do not toss the animal to the floor the moment your mission is accomplished. Not only can this make future pill-giving a major problem, but your cat is likely to give you the cold shoulder for weeks. Give him a reward afterward, some dry food or a teaspoon of canned food.

Pilling a Difficult Cat

Some cats can not be fooled and must be restrained in order to get their medication. Wrap the animal in a towel from the neck down, making sure his paws are securely encased, then force open his mouth and proceed as described above.

Cautions, Reminders, and Tips

- Always coat pills with some sort of oil, butter or soft fat.
- If your cat begins to cough or gag, the pill might have gotten into his windpipe. Release his mouth immediately so the pill can be coughed up. If it isn't coughed up, you can help dislodge it by holding the cat upside down—and call your veterinarian!
- If there's no way your cat will swallow a pill, turn the medication into a liquid and administer it with a plastic (not glass) eyedropper. Fill the dropper with a solution of crushed pill mixed with a beaten raw yolk and a teaspoon, or so, of Karo syrup. Gently push the dropper between your pet's lips. If he tries to bite the dropper, the act will cause him to swallow. If this procedure doesn't work, you can try tilting the animal's head, just slightly, and administering the medicine slowly, making sure the medicine does not enter the windpipe. If your cat begins to cough or gag, stop immediately.
- Another alternative for medicating zealous pill-protesters is to mix the crushed pill with an extremely appetizing, odor-masking food. Oil-packed sardines are your best bet—unless FLUTD is a problem, in which case sardines, high in magnesium, are a no-no. Forget trying to mix a crushed pill into your pet's regular food; a cat's nose knows.

Q&A

Harried About Hair Balls

My three-year-old Birman grooms herself frequently and is constantly distressed by hair balls. She's not what I would describe as a willing patient, and it's always a struggle to get medication down. Are there any foods she should eat that would lessen her hair loss, and do you have any suggestions for easy hair-ball medicine administration?

My first suggestion is that you begin grooming her more often, which should decrease some of the hair she's ingesting. My next suggestion is to be sure she's receiving high-BV protein and fat in her diet, a good daily supplement, and perhaps a vegetable enzyme. This, along with a humidifier in your home, should help minimize her shedding. As for administering hair-ball medicine, the simplest way is to buy a product such as Petromalt or Laxatone and put a fingerful on her nose or toes; she'll ingest it as she licks it off, or add Booda Mix to her food.

Getting Your Cat to Do What You Want Him to Do

I know that my cat is suffering from poor nutrition. He has a dull coat, cracked pads, an eye discharge and simply doesn't play like he used to. His veterinarian says that he has to eat a professional/alternative food, but he simply won't! I love him so much, what can I do?

If you don't get him to eat a balanced diet he is going to become susceptible to disease and will get very sick. You are smarter and bigger than he is, so let's remember that. Mix a tiny portion of quality food that you "think he might like," canned or dry (you decide based on his current preference). If you are feeding him just people food, simply add a small amount of the balanced food every day, increasing little by little. You may never get him to eat 100% cat food, but 95% would make a big difference for both of you!

Is My Cat Bulimic?

He eats and then vomits almost all the time. Does he need a behaviorist?

No, he needs to slow down and be less nervous. If you are feeding dry food, get a big rock, wash it and place it in the middle of the food. That's going to slow him down significantly.

Pet him as he eats. Add chamomile tea (1/8 teaspoon) and vegetable enzyme to his canned food to help digestion.

Lastly, if he is eating with other cats, separate him. Maybe he won't try to be the fastest eater.

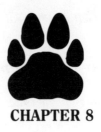

CHAPTER 8

....

Getting Emotional

....

Bad Behavior
*The more you know about a cat, the less trouble
you'll have with him.*

I've never met a bad cat, but quite a few brought to me are described as such. Not, I must admit, without reason. They're usually aggressive—biters, fighters, dauntless troublemakers with unpleasant personalities and obnoxious habits. On occasion they're spiteful introverts with mouselike machismo and the charisma of soggy cornflakes.

The first idea I try to convey to the owner is that it is the cat's behavior, not the cat itself, that is bad. What's the difference, you might ask (as many owners do). A big one! If the cause of unsocial or abnormal behavior can be determined, there's a chance of correcting it.

A "bad" cat is a victim: All *"bad"* cats are the unwitting victims of circumstances beyond their control, but not necessarily beyond that of their owners. Although it's true that certain undesirable traits are inherited, these can be controlled and even eliminated, if the kitten is taken at four weeks and hand-raised. Unfortunately, this is not always possible. Therefore, I advise owners to find out as much as they can about a queen before picking a pet from her litter. To my mind, it's criminal for anyone to breed an overly nervous, aggressive, hyperactive, extremely timid or otherwise genetically undesirable cat; yet, regrettably, people continue to do so.

Nevertheless, it's environment, not heredity, that molds most cats' behavior—and the person responsible for the ambience that surrounds a cat is you!

Problems, Possible Causes, and Nutritional Remedies

Feeding your cat for better behavior

Behavioral problems in cats have many possible causes. Because some problems are often symptoms or side effects of injury or disease, none can be ignored. It's important, therefore, to consult a veterinarian who has examined your cat and knows his medical history BEFORE you make any of the dietary changes that I suggest here and throughout the book.

Aggression

SYMPTOMS: Biting, scratching, active hostility

POSSIBLE CAUSES: Early subjection to abuse or indifference; impaired vision; brain tumor; inner-ear infection; any infection or pain; fear; environmental stress (a move, a new baby or pet in the household); domestic tension; maternal protectiveness

FOR YOUR INFORMATION: It is not normal for a cat to bite and scratch its owners, household members, or friends; sudden, unprovoked attacks should be brought to a veterinarian's attention. Train your cat as a kitten that biting is not allowed; you can do so by gently countering a nip with a quick finger-flick to the nose and a firm "no," while continuing to pet him. Foods rich in niacin (as well as all the B vitamins), brewer's or torula yeast, are highly recommended for calming rambunctious little Rambos. Exercise and love are essential. The Laser Kat is a great exercise product. For more information about the Laser Kat call 313-538-7333.

SUGGESTED
NUTRITIONAL
REMEDY:

- Discontinue feeding any supermarket/ commercial food with artificial coloring or more than one preservative. Absolutely no soft-moist food should be offered.
- Add 1/4 teaspoon of brewer's yeast or torula yeast to food daily.
- Add 1 teaspoon of chamomile tea three times daily, mixed with food or administered as described in chapter 7.
- Add 2–3 drops Bach Rescue Remedy to water or food daily.
- Replace 2 tablespoons regular food with 2 tablespoons finely chopped, cooked white-meat turkey (no skin) three to five times weekly.
- Give 1/4 cup warm milk before bedtime.
- Add ground hops to food.

Shyness

SYMPTOMS: Frightened, nervous, timid, hides

POSSIBLE
CAUSES: Insufficient physical contact with people or other animals; inherited nervousness; shock reaction to a frightening or painful experience (fight, explosion, sudden injury, surgery) or a narrow escape from one; early abandonment; central nervous system disorder; thyroid malfunction; gastrointestinal discomfort; overeating; any illness or pain.

FOR YOUR
INFORMATION: Unless shyness is genetically inherited, timidity in cats most commonly results from being raised in either a very noisy or a very cloistered environment, or from having either extremely anxious or totally indifferent owners. Gastrointestinal upsets

are common among shy and nervous cats, so you should make a special effort to supply easily digestible food and extra, stress fighting B vitamins. Exercise and love are essential. The Laser Kat is one of the best exercise products available. For more information about the Laser Kat call 313-538-7333.

SUGGESTED NUTRITIONAL REMEDY:

- Feed at least twice daily and allow free feeding. Feed meals in a quiet area, away from other pets or children.
- Leave dry food down all day long (diet food if your cat is overweight). Make sure the food is in a quiet, safe place so he can nibble when it seems safe.
- Feed regular meals in a quiet place, away from the general household traffic.
- Add 1/4–1/2 teaspoon brewer's or torula yeast to the food daily, or give it as a treat.
- Add 1/4 teaspoon chamomile tea to the food to help calm and digest.
- Provide large portions of TLC, interactive play (such as blowing soap bubbles), and regular daily petting, and/or gentle grooming in a SAFE, QUIET place.
- Add 2–3 drops of Bach Flower Rescue Remedy or Homeopet Anti-Anxiety Drops to the food or water.
- Give an antioxidant.

Neurotic Behavior

SYMPTOMS: Eating wool, fabrics, or feces; tail chewing

POSSIBLE CAUSES: Lack of companionship and attention; dietary deficiency of vitamins, minerals, fiber, or digestive enzymes; worms; confinement; insufficient mental and physical stimulation; nonspecific illness or pain

FOR YOUR INFORMATION: Wool and fabric eating, generally stemming from the frustrations of boredom, confinement, or inattention, is common among indoor cats whose diets are deficient primarily in fiber. Siamese-type breeds are known for their love of fabric. Feces eating appears in cats with equivalent nutritional deficiencies, often caused by a perpetual cycling of intestinal parasites. Tail chewers are mostly feline versions of depressed, attention-deprived, thumb suckers and nail-biters. Owner enlightenment, in conjunction with nutrient supplementation, has proven enormously successful in eliminating these related problems. Prozac,™ Elavil,™ and other drugs of their class are often prescribed for those cats that don't respond to other therapies.

• Give 1/4–1/2 cup warm milk with honey
(serve when it is room temperature).

Exercise and love are essential. The Laser Kat is a great exercise product. For more information about the Laser Kat call 313-538-7333.

SUGGESTED NUTRITIONAL REMEDY:

• If you are not feeding a professional/ alternative food that includes beet pulp, whole grains, bran or some other fiber, substitute 1 teaspoon of any one of these: canned green beans, lima beans, grated, raw carrots, or peas, for an equal portion of your cat's regular food.
• Leave dry food down all day long (diet food if your cat is overweight). Make sure the food is in a quiet, safe place, so he can nibble when it seems safe.
• Check the fiber percentage. You may want to change to a food with higher fiber.
• Add 1/8 teaspoon brewer's or torula yeast once a day to meals.
• Add 1/8 teaspoon of bran.
• Grow wheat grass for your cat to chew on.
• Add 1/4 teaspoon chamomile tea to food twice daily.

- Let your cat play with catnip; it might seem to get him "high," but he will settle down afterward.
- Provide lots of TLC and playful activity.

Forgetting Housebreaking

SYMPTOMS: Spraying, ignoring the litter box, soiling floors and furniture

POSSIBLE
CAUSES: Hostility; urinary infection (cystitis); kidney disease; old age; illness; recuperation after surgery or illness; food dish and littler box too close to one another; spinal injury; head injury; emotional stress; unclean litter box; needs to be neutered; jealousy; new cats outside.

FOR YOUR
INFORMATION: Cats, under normal circumstances, are naturally fastidious and easily trained to use a litter box, but an infrequently cleaned litter box, or one with scented litter, can break their training. Urination in other household areas is often a symptom of cystitis (which causes painful, frequent voiding), or the result, after recovery, of having become habituated to not using the litter box. Geriatric cats frequently lose control of bladder and bowel function. Emotional stress, which can be caused by dietary as well as environmental changes, is generally the cause of voiding and defecating on furniture.

- Clean the litter box with a product that is non-toxic and that does not leave an odor that could be noxious to the cat.
- Clean the areas where the inappropriate urination or defecation is occurring with an enzymatic cleaner.
- Provide attention and activity (particularly for toms and neutered males) to prevent boredom

and frustration, which are often the cause of indoor spraying.

Exercise and love are essential. The Laser Kat is an excellent exercise product. For more information about the Laser Kat call 313-538-7333.

SUGGESTED NUTRITIONAL REMEDY:

- Feed only quality, high-BV-protein (low magnesium) food that produces an acidic urine. Please allow free feeding.
- Add 1/8–1/4 teaspoon brewer's or torula yeast, once a day, to meals.
- Give 100–200 mg of vitamin C.
- Mix 1–2 teaspoons tomato juice into canned food three to five times weekly.
- Supply plenty of water. Hard water contains magnesium, so I'd suggest you provide noncarbonated, bottled water at room temperature and keep it fresh daily.
- Keep the food dish and the litter box in separate areas. (You wouldn't want to dine in your bathroom, would you?)
- Give your cat antianxiety remedy by homeopet as per directions on the package.

Q&A

Maine Coon Maniac

I have a large, four-year-old Maine Coon who has turned into a destructive maniac. His name is Jack, and I've taken to calling him Jack the Ripper because of the way he's clawed up the house. My couch and draperies are ruined, but I'm not buying new ones until I can get Jack under control. He has a scratching post and behaves when I'm around, but when I go to work, so does he—on everything. I'd hate to have him declawed, but I don't know what else to do. Help!

I would combine a behavioral approach with a nutritional one. Buy Jack a scratching tunnel, or cylinder, something he can play and hide in. Spray it with catnip and place it next to his favorite (i.e., the couch). Play with him in his carpeted play area. When you see him scratch in the wrong places, hit some place close with a rolled up section of a newspaper. This will make noise and frighten him. Don't talk, because then he will know it's you, and he probably could care less. Then bring him to his new place and put his paws on it.

Play with him at scheduled times so he can look forward to it— play anything he likes.

I would add torula or brewer's yeast to his food along with chamomile tea (start with 1–3 drops, and add more daily). Try to work up to 1 teaspoon in each meal. Keep him away from any food with artificial coloring, preservatives, or sugar. You can leave dry food down all day (use diet dry food, if he is chubby).

Plastic Bags Anyone?

My cat loves to eat plastic bags—in fact, anything plastic. He also licks the cement floor in the basement. I feed him canned food and give him people food from time to time. What should I do?

Let's start by removing all plastic. Next, let's make sure he is eating a professional/alternative dry food with some type of fiber. If he insists on eating canned food, then it, too, should be professional/ alternative, but add a mixture of oat bran and torula yeast (1 part each) to his food. Start with 1/8 teaspoon of this fiber/yeast mixture, going up to 1/4 teaspoon.

I also want you to add Prozyme to his food or Dr. Jane® Beezyme. This will ensure that most of the nutrients from the food will be digested.

If he continues to lick the cement floor, there is nothing to do except make sure it's clean and free of heavy-duty cleaning detergents.

The Night Howler

My Siamese keeps me up from 3 A.M. until dawn—he howls all over the apartment. What do I do? I've tried tranquilizers, but he still howls; it's just not as strong.

Let's play with him before bedtime. Try to tire him out. Also give him hot milk and honey just before you go to bed, leaving dry food for him to nibble all night.

During the day, add some brewer's or torula yeast to his food. The B vitamins in the yeast may help him calm down a little. You can also add 1–3 drops of chamomile tea to his water every day and/or Homeopet Anti-Anxiety Drops.

Remember, Siamese like to talk; it's just unfortunate that he has chosen the middle of the night to express himself. Hopefully, all of the above will keep his conversation to a minimum.

CHAPTER 9

. . . .

Getting Territorial

. . . .

The Indoor Cat

*Easily satisfied and easily cared for, his special needs
can be too easily ignored.*

Some cats are more suited than others to the indoor life, but virtually all can become conditioned to it. The conditioning process is not difficult, provided you understand that cats are inherently territorial, are creatures of habit, have unique nutritional needs, and their natural instincts don't disappear just because they've been raised on canned prey, in a world of wall-to-wall carpeting.

Pitfalls of Raising an Indoor Cat: The needs of indoor cats are often misunderstood by well-meaning owners who tend to lavish food on their pets as a demonstration of affection, unknowingly defeating their purpose by setting up the animals they love for a major fall from health. Limited space provides limited room for activity. Limited activity, plus unlimited calories, adds pounds and sums up obesity, decreasing the cat's life expectancy and increasing his chances for an unpleasant assortment of ailments.

Another common pitfall is allowing the cat to dictate his own diet ("Oh, Mommy's poor baby's been alone all day, so I'll give her anything she wants"), which usually winds up being a single food, or type of food, which excludes all others. You can not only create a finicky eater, but also a powerful food addiction. So powerful is this addiction, that if at any future time a prescription diet becomes a life-or-death necessity, the cat might only be capable of opting for the second choice.

Feeding for Close Quarters: The best foods for any cat, providing he has no specially prescribed dietary restrictions, are those with the highest protein/fat digestibility and utilization. These foods not only supply optimal nutrition, but also produce fewer and less odorous stools, which, let's face it, is a definite plus for anyone living with a cat in a small apartment.

Health Memos: Because they are deprived of seasonal, natural light, and temperature cycles, which influence shedding, most indoor cats shed year-round. They are, therefore, more prone to hair balls and likely to need hair-ball medication at least once or twice a week. Grooming is necessary, even for shorthairs, since their environment does not provide the tall-grass, natural brushing available to outdoor cats.

Offer your indoor cat opportunities for as much exercise play as possible. If you're too busy to interact with your pet, a paper bag (for pouncing on, crawling in and out of, batting around) and/or a rubber ball, can keep an indoor cat amused and active for quite a while.

Luckily, all cat foods have more than enough vitamin D, since indoor cats are denied the benefits of the sun. I suggest a "vita light," which supplies some of the rays your cat simply isn't getting inside. Cats love to lie under the heat and with this full-spectrum light, all they need is Bain de Soleil!

The Outdoor Cat

The more territory he roams, the greater his health hazards.

An outdoor cat is not necessarily one who lives outdoors, but (at least for the purposes of this book) one who has the freedom and opportunity to spend a substantial amount of unsupervised time outside the confines of his home. Whether you put your cat out at night, or let him in, the hours your pet spends on his own—and the way he spends them—definitely affect his physical and emotional well-being.

Dangerous Assumptions About Outdoor Cats: Because felines are natural outdoor survivalists, many owners assume their cat will instinctively take care of himself, as well as cure his own ailments, if allowed enough time outside. Well, from my veterinary experience, let me tell you that this just ain't so. Once a cat is outdoors, he is going to follow his instincts, and these are what most often lead to trouble. Outdoor cats can get into fights with cats and other animals, come into contact with poisons, get hit by cars, stuck in traps, or stuck inside buildings, just to name a few dangers. Carnivorous and predatory, a cat, no matter what you feed it, will rarely pass up the chance to bring down an unwary bird or rodent. Even if that prey is not eaten, but just brought to your door with a proud "meow," it's highly unlikely that your cat won't eventually want a taste of his catch, and invariably ingest more than desired. Two words of caution: internal parasites; these can be very dangerous.

Cats with well-fortified immune systems are more resistant to the debilitating effects of worms (intestinal parasites), which can be contracted rather easily. A healthy immune system is a must for outdoor felines, who are more susceptible to contagious viral and bacterial infections because of the increased possibility of contact with sick strays and access to contaminated food or water.

Health Memos: If your pet is a four-footed nature lover, I strongly recommend feeding a daily diet of high-BV-protein, vitamin-enriched professional/alternative food, supplemented with 1/4 teaspoon of brewer's or torula yeast and 100–200 mg of vitamin C with fresh garlic daily.

Before letting a kitten or cat outside, be sure he has received all essential inoculations (distemper, rhino-tracheitis, pneumonitis, calici-virus, rabies) and any required annual booster shots.

The Multi-Cat Home

When there's more than one, don't double the problems, double the fun.

Cats, by nature, are solitary animals, but, by golly, they can enjoy company. Not all cats, of course, and not all the time . . . and not always the companions we choose for them. Nonetheless, as every cat lover knows, once you're hooked on one, there will usually be another (if not more) in your future—and in your home—a lot sooner than you think.

Coping Simplified: When you're dealing with cats, proper introductions have nothing to do with etiquette and everything to do with establishing peace (or at least détente), and keeping your sanity intact.

Prior to bringing home the new, soon-to-be-permanent guest, dab inexpensive perfume or talc on the new guest and on your own cat(s). It helps when every cat smells the same.

If the new arrival is a kitten, speak softly, handle gently, and put him in a quiet room away from your resident pet (and children). Provide fresh water, food, a litter pan and a soft resting place. Allow the kitten to investigate his new surroundings at his own pace. Your resident pet will be curious about the intruder, but for the first few days do not leave them alone together. Hostility is natural and can be hazardous to a kitten's health. Don't forget to cut the nails on both cats. The two will soon establish a relationship. Giving your older cat some extra affection during this period will help make that relationship a friendlier one.

If you bring in an adult cat, plan on postponing pet introductions for at least five days. This newcomer will usually be heavily stressed and behaviorally unpredictable. He needs adjustment time in an off-limits living space of his own, in order to feel secure and come to trust you. Patience in this situation is not just a virtue, it's a necessity for communal cat comfort.

Health Memos: Extra attention and B vitamins (either brewer's or torula yeast or 50–75 mg of B complex) and 100 mg of vitamin C (50 mg for kittens) should be given to the new cat, as well as your resident pet during this period, and for at least two weeks after they've been introduced. Homeopet Anti-Anxiety Remedy—or catnip tea for the older cat and/or crushed hops mixed with the food—will certainly decrease anxiety.

Each cat should have his own feeding dish. If either cat begins vomiting after meals, which is often caused by competitive eating (rapid gobbling of food), feed them in different areas or at different times.

Be sure any new cat you bring home has been fully inoculated and tested for communicable diseases before introducing him to your resident pets.

When Cats Live with Other Animals

How to keep purrr-fect harmony in an interspecies household

Whether a cat shares his home with dogs, hamsters, birds, snakes, guinea pigs, parakeets or kids, it still needs a place to call his own and will usually find and claim it all by himself. The myth that dogs and cats are natural adversaries is just that: a myth. In domestic situations, animals aren't born enemies, they're made. And once you realize that any multi-pet home can run as smoothly as Noah's ark with a little common sense, consistent rules, and the word "no," you've got it made.

Avoiding Mealtime Mayhem: Food is really the only problem, especially if any of your pets happen to be natural feline fare. A new cat entering a home that has a resident bird or gerbil, shouldn't be expected to know that these are its neighbors and not its larder. But it can learn. It's easy enough to teach a kitten by squirting it with water from a toy water pistol any time he even approaches those animals' cages, but older cats can be more difficult to dissuade. For them, I'd suggest keeping your smaller, ingestible pets secured in rooms that the cat is never allowed to enter. And I do mean never. Even the sweetest, gentlest cat in the world is capable of taking a lethal swipe at a small, caged creature, so boundaries must be firmly established and precautions taken.

As for regular feedings of cats and dogs in the same household, the important idea to remember is that they need separate dining areas or different eating times. Most dogs adore cat food, and since they're also prone to competitive eating, they often scarf down their own meal and then go for the cat's. If you're unaware of this, you may find your cat inexplicably losing weight, always appearing hungry, and possibly convince yourself (and even your vet) that there's a medical problem, when in fact it's a canine problem. On the other hand, cats will often eat dog food, which is deficient in taurine (essential for felines) and can become too full to eat their own nutritious dinners.

Health Memos: Supervise dog and cat mealtimes, and do not leave food down all day for either animal.

Never serve more than one animal from the same feeding dish.

Add brewer's yeast or torula yeast to both the cat and dog's food daily. A little stress prevention never hurts.

If one animal has worms, the others should be checked for them, since they are commonly transmitted between cats and dogs.

Keep track of inoculations and yearly booster shots. Even if your cat doesn't leave the house, your dog most likely does and can bring home big trouble. Fleas are also easy to share.

Conjunctivitis, an inflammation of the tissues surrounding the eye, can be transmitted from dog to cat and vice versa. Although not all types of conjunctivitis are contagious, it's best to quarantine the afflicted pet until you get an okay from your vet.

Changing Your Cat's Environment

When a cat is moved from one environment to another, a right diet might turn out to be all wrong.

A move is never easy for anyone, but it's especially difficult for cats. Whether you're taking your pet south for the winter, or bringing him up north to a friend, there are emotional and nutritional considerations that should be kept in mind.

Right Moves: When your cat arrives at the new home, do not expect him to behave as usual. This is all new territory for the animal, unfamiliar turf, and no matter how lovely the new environment, your cat is not going to be thrilled.

If you're used to letting your pet outdoors, do not do so unless there is a fenced-in area, or unless you walk him on a leash for at least two weeks. As remarkable as cats are for finding their way home, it will take a while for them to get

> DOGS CAN EAT CAT FOOD, BUT THEY MAY GET FAT AND GET DIARRHEA. CATS CAN'T EAT DOG FOOD. THERE IS NOT ENOUGH PROTEIN, FAT OR TAURINE!

used to a new one. And if they don't like the new home, they just might try to hightail it back to their old home.

If you're leaving your cat with a friend, bring along some of your pet's familiar things (toys, bed, feeding dish, the pillow case you used the night before), and be sure to have your friend keep the animal's regular feeding schedule and diet. Adding 50–75 mg B complex and 100 mg vitamin C to the food will help reduce stress, and replacing a fourth of the cat's first few meals with a favorite treat meat or protein will soften the blow of staying with a stranger. Be sure to keep your cat's regular feeding routine. Even if you don't usually leave dry food down, leave some down for a while—your cat may be too upset to eat until he wants to do so.

Health Memos: Antioxidants should be started at least 2 weeks before the move.

Brewer's or Torula yeast should also be included in the food.

1–3 drops of Bach Rescue Remedy or chamomile tea should be added to the water about one week prior to leaving, and continued in the new environment until your cat feels secure.

Lots of TLC is needed at specific times. Since shedding may increase because of fear, combing and brushing is a must. Hair-ball remedy every other day (unless your cat has loose stools) is also a good idea because some cats get constipated under stress.

Q&A

The Boy Next Door

A new neighborhood panhandler (unaltered male cat) has recently moved to my area. My cats, female and male, are acting strange. One of them is urinating on the window sill, while the other is going around the house screaming! My little female cat refuses to eat and won't let me play with her. Help!

The first thing I would do is find the cat's owner and have that cat altered! We have enough unwanted cats in the street. The urine you are finding on the window sill is probably from your cat marking his territory. Wash that area with an enzymatic cleaner that will get rid of all smell and spray it daily with a repellent.

Your cats definitely need anti-stress nutrition. Try brewer's or torula yeast, 1/4 teaspoon per cat, in each meal. I would sprinkle a little hops on their food as well and give them catnip to play with daily.

Part Four

· ·

Dr. Jane's New-Life Nutrition Plan

· ·

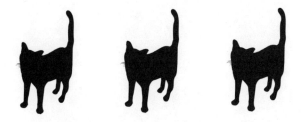

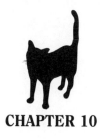

CHAPTER 10

. . . .

Thirty Days to a Healthier and Happier Cat

. . . .

I have designed the 30-day regimen so that it will be easy for you and your cat to comply. The month is divided into four weeks. I ask you to evaluate your cat at the beginning of the four weeks and then at the end of every week, so that you can see how well you are both doing.

The evaluation is easy. It includes physical appearance, bodily functions (urination, defecation), and behavior. You will evaluate your cat using a score from 1 to 3, with 3 being the healthiest score and 1 being the least healthy. If your cat starts with a 1 or 2, you will see it change to a 3 by the end of the 30 days.

Knowing cats are creatures of habit, and don't like change, I have structured the weeks to be similar to each other. It is important that you are comfortable with the daily regimen from the first week, so that your cat gets used to the changes and even welcomes them. You will see that the weekly continuity allows you to develop a routine that makes the 30-day plan simple to use and EFFECTIVE.

My afternoon recipes are NOT balanced—they are only afternoon treats— if you choose, you may add powdered egg shell to them all. Take an egg—use it for something else, and save the egg shell. Mash the shell as best you can. It must be cooked or sauteed.

How to Evaluate Your Cat for the 30-Day Diet

- *Physical Appearance—close up and far away*

- *Bodily Functions*

- *Behavior*

#1: Looking at your cat from a distance

A) Does he have a waist line?
(a slight tuck right in front of the knees)
- ☐ A grossly overweight cat is round
   with no tuck in sight   GRADE 1
- ☐ An overweight cat has a slight tuck   GRADE 2
- ☐ A cat with the correct weight has a
   noticeable tuck   GRADE 3

B) Does his stomach touch the ground?
- ☐ Stomach touches the ground   GRADE 1
- ☐ Stomach loose, but off the ground   GRADE 2
- ☐ Stomach tucked in—tightly   GRADE 3

#2: Looking at your cat close up

Place your cat on a table, with its head away from you.
You will evaluate the cat from nose to tail.

A) Are his whiskers long and full?
- ☐ Short, sparse whiskers   GRADE 1
- ☐ Full, long whiskers   GRADE 2
- ☐ Very full and long whiskers   GRADE 3
   (very difficult to grade—may want to compare with
   another cat)

B) Are his eyes free of discharge?
- ☐ A discharge every day that can be white, yellow, or brown   **GRADE 1**
- ☐ A slight discharge that isn't necessarily daily that can be white, yellow, or watery   **GRADE 2**
- ☐ No discharge   **GRADE 3**
  (some breeds of cats normally have discharge; Persian, Burmese, Himalayan)

C) Does his breath smell?
- ☐ A foul smell (not caused by diet)   **GRADE 1**
- ☐ A slight smell   **GRADE 2**
- ☐ No smell   **GRADE 3**

D) What is his coat like?
- ☐ Dull and/or brittle and/or thin, noticeably dull, or has sores   **GRADE 1**
- ☐ Relatively full, a little dry, or brittle, or thin with no sores   **GRADE 2**
- ☐ Thick, full, shiny coat—no sores   **GRADE 3**

E) What is his skin like?
- ☐ Very flaky, dandruff, red and irritated in places. When you feel with your finger there is a lot of oil, or absolutely no oil at all   **GRADE 1**
- ☐ Some flakes, dandruff, no sores on the body, your finger feels oily or dry   **GRADE 2**
- ☐ No flakes, no dandruff, no sores; your finger detects only a slight film   **GRADE 3**

F) Is it clean around the area of the tail?
- ☐ Feces, or dirt on the hair   **GRADE 1**
- ☐ A little dirty, but relatively clean   **GRADE 2**
- ☐ Clean   **GRADE 3**

G) Length and condition of his nails and pads?
- ☐ Short, brittle nails and/or dry, cracked pads (if an outdoor cat, the pads will be thicker than indoor, but should not be cracked)   **GRADE 1**
- ☐ Short, and/or brittle nails, with dry pads   **GRADE 2**
- ☐ Long healthy nails, soft pads   **GRADE 3**

H)   Feel for his ribs by placing one hand on the left shoulder, the other hand on the right shoulder.
     Moving toward the tail, do you feel ribs?
     ☐ Ribs may be there, but you can't really feel them, or they are VERY PROMINENT   **GRADE 1**
     ☐ Ribs are there, but under more than a pinch of fat   **GRADE 2**
     ☐ Ribs are there, with just a pinch of fat   **GRADE 3**

#3: Bodily Functions

A)   **What is his appetite like?**
     ☐ Appetite is unusual; ravenous or none at all   **GRADE 1**
     ☐ Appetite is almost normal   **GRADE 2**
     ☐ Appetite is the same as it usually is   **GRADE 3**

B)   **Are there digestive problems?**
     ☐ Hair balls, regurgitation, vomiting
       more than one time daily   **GRADE 1**
     ☐ Hair balls, regurgitation, vomiting daily   **GRADE 2**
     ☐ No hair balls, regurgitation or vomiting   **GRADE 3**

C)   **What is the condition of the stool?**
     ☐ Stools are odorous, loose and/or voluminous
       and occur more than two times daily   **GRADE 1**
     ☐ Stools are slightly odorous, slightly loose
       and occur once or twice daily   **GRADE 2**
     ☐ Stools are odorless, or just slightly odorous,
       firm, and occur once or twice daily   **GRADE 3**

#4: Behavior

A)   **How is his activity?**
     ☐ Activity decreased, sluggish, or irritable and
       stays alone   **GRADE 1**
     ☐ Activity may be normal or slightly decreased,
       and may be a little irritable   **GRADE 2**
     ☐ Activity and personality are normal   **GRADE 3**

Kitten (until 1 year old)

This is the beginning of the work week for many of us. The kitten living on the "weekend" schedule with its less demanding pace, now has to adjust to the long work days. Even if the primary caretaker doesn't go to work on Monday, the kitten can feel there is a difference in life style—trust me! The following weekly guide will reflect these living changes.

M O N D A Y

A.M.

- 1/2 can (6 oz.) or one (3 oz.) can kitten food

- 1/8 teaspoon Dr. Jane® Beezyme

- 1/4 cup professional/ alternative dry kitten food just before you leave

The food should be a professional/alternative food. This is a critical developmental time.

It's a good idea to avoid fish foods since some can be high in magnesium, and some adult cats may need to avoid them. You can select any flavor you like, just don't change the brand of food.

Use Dr. Jane® Beezyme, but if it is not available, mix bee pollen with a vegetable enzyme. If you have not used it before, then just put a slight sprinkle on the food, increasing the amount daily until you arrive at 1/8 teaspoonful. Mix food well.

Put down dry kitten food just before you leave. The brand can be different from the canned food, but make sure you stick with the brand of dry food you select.

comment . . . *If your kitten does not finish the canned food before you leave, I would pick it up and refrigerate it. Use it for the evening meal, but be sure to warm it up.*

Early

P.M.

- Yogurt mixed with a sprinkle of dry kitten food

- Comb/groom

- Exercise

- Antioxidant

You can select any type of yogurt, with or without fruit, as long as it contains "live cultures." The amount will vary with the activity of your kitten, ranging from 1–3 tablespoons of yogurt mixed with 1/8 cup of dry food.

Make sure that your brush is appropriate, not too soft, not too hard. Brush backward from tail to head, then go from head to tail. During flea season, use a flea comb and comb your kitten from head to tail. Throw dead hair and flea dirt in the toilet.

KITTY TEASE

Use a kitty tease or a long pole with a feather or sock. Let the kitten run, jump and chase it for as long as you both can last!

Use Dr. Jane® Feline Formula One or another antioxidant.

comment . . . *The yogurt contains bacteria necessary for a healthy intestinal tract. Feeding, brushing/combing, and playing with your cat will help develop that special bond you want from your cat. Brushing or combing helps eliminate hair balls and promotes healthy skin and coat.*

DINNER

- 1/2 can (6 oz.) or one (3 oz.) can kitten food
- 1/8 teaspoon Dr. Jane® Beezyme

Warm the leftover food with hot water (small amount), or place the food in the microwave for 3 seconds, stirring it before you serve!

comment . . . *If your kitten doesn't want to eat all its food, you can leave it down for a few hours. Sometimes a kitten is so busy playing, it simply forgets it's dinnertime. (If your kitten is not eating and is not playing, call your family veterinarian.)*

BEFORE BED

- Exercise
- Clean teeth
- Hair-ball medicine
- Warm milk and honey
- 1/8–1/4 cup professional/ alternative dry food for the evening
- Liver treats

Exercise using the same toy you did earlier in the evening.

Cleaning teeth: hold your kitten on a table or counter. Face its head away from you, the tail toward you. Take a toothbrush made for a kitten, or a finger cot, add toothpaste and brush your kitten's back teeth. After you do one side, reward him with love, then do the other side. It will get easier every day you do it. Just do one side once—if you didn't do a good-enough job, you will do better tomorrow.

Hair-ball medicine: Offer him one squeeze of a hair-ball medicine. If he won't lick it, put it on his nose or toes—it will be licked soon enough!

Heat 1/4–1/2 cup of milk with 1/8 teaspoonful of honey. Make sure it does not boil, that it is luke warm.

Once you know your kitten's appetite better, you will know how much food to give.

comment . . . *It's important to get your kitten used to being handled, especially to clean its teeth. Make the experience as pleasant as you can. You can reward your kitten with a small amount of kitten food or with Dr. Jane's liver treats.*

Dr. Jane's Liver Treats

1 cup flour	1/2 cup wheat germ
1 cup cornmeal	1 lb. raw, organic beef or lamb liver
1/4 teaspoon chopped, fresh garlic	1 pinch of salt

Put liver in blender or food processor to liquefy it. (You may want to cut it into small pieces before you blend it.)

Add the above ingredients, mixing well.

Grease a cookie sheet. Place 1 large teaspoonful of mixture in rows on the cookie sheet. Flatten the patties with the bottom of a glass dipped in corn meal. Bake at 350° for 15–20 minutes.

TUESDAY

A.M.

- 1/2 can (6 oz.) or one (3 oz.) can kitten food
- 1/8 teaspoon Dr. Jane® Beezyme
- 1/4 cup professional/ alternative dry kitten food just before you leave.

The flavor can be different from Monday, but the manufacturer must be the same.

Keep adding more Beezyme® if you are not up to 1/8 teaspoon yet.

Use the same type of dry kitten food as you did on Monday. You can leave more if your kitten was hungry yesterday when you got home.

comment . . . *You may want to alter the amount of food you give in the morning. If your kitten wants more canned food, and is not getting fat, add a little more.*

Early P.M.

- 1–2 tablespoons cheese
- 1/8 cup professional/ alternative dry kitten food
- Comb/groom
- Exercise
- Antioxidant

Ricotta cheese, or cottage cheese sprinkled with dry kitten food.

Don't forget to brush the wrong way first.

ALUMINUM BALL

Make a ball about the size of a quarter and throw it. The ball is light enough to be picked up in his mouth. You can buy foam rubber balls which are also great to play with. Throw the ball, let your kitten go after it, and then try to get him to bring it back to you. If that fails, make 6–10 balls, throwing them one by one, making your kitten run after them.

DINNER

- 1/2 can (6 oz.) or one (3 oz.) can kitten food
- 1/8 teaspoon Dr. Jane® Beezyme

Remember not to serve cold food.

Use the same amount of Dr. Jane® Beezyme you did in the morning if you are not up to 1/8 teaspoonful yet.

BEFORE BED

- Exercise
- Clean teeth
- Warm milk and honey
- 1/8–1/4 cup professional/ alternative dry food for the evening

If your kitten is very playful, you may want to throw 20 balls. The object is to tire the kitten out, or at least use a lot of his energy so you can sleep at night.

Heat 1/4–1/2 cup of milk with 1/8 teaspoonful of honey. Make sure it does not boil; serve it luke-warm.

Don't forget to leave out his dry food.

comment . . . *If you wake up and find there is dry food left over, you will leave less tomorrow night. Your kitten may not require the additional food during the night.*

W E D N E S D A Y

A.M.

- 1/2 can (6 oz.) or one (3 oz.) can kitten food
- 1/8 teaspoon Dr. Jane® Beezyme
- Leave 1/4 cup professional/ alternative dry kitten food just before you leave.

You can use a different flavor but not a different brand.

You should be adding more Dr. Jane® Beezyme than yesterday, until you get to 1/8 teaspoon.

If you find that your kitten was hungry when you got home yesterday, then you can increase this to 1/2 cup.

comment . . . *By this time you should be getting into an easy routine.*

Early

P.M.

- Kitten Left-Over Casserole
- Comb/groom
- Exercise
- Antioxidant

Kitten Left-Over Casserole

2 tablespoons chopped cooked meat	1/8 cup of dry kitten food
1/4 teaspoonful minced cooked vegetables	

Mix 2 tablespoons of chopped, cooked meat with 1/4 teaspoonful of minced, cooked vegetable (it does not have to be reheated) with 1/8 cup of dry kitten food.

Early P.M.

- Exercise

STRING & BAG

Take a 2–3-inch-wide cord, about 8 feet long. Tie the end into a fat knot. Take a paper bag and place it in the middle of a room, with the knot inside the bag. Step away, holding the string, and slowly pull it out of the bag as your cat chases it. Kittens and cats love the noise of a paper bag!

comment . . . *This time of the day is very important to your cat. Chances are, you just got home from work, and the kitten was all alone. The kitten is lonely and wants to be with its owner.*

DINNER

- 1/2 can (6 oz.) or one (3 oz.) can kitten food
- 1/8 teaspoon Dr. Jane® Beezyme

Remember not to serve cold food.

You should be increasing the amount slowly until you reach 1/8 teaspoon.

BEFORE BED

- Exercise
- Clean teeth
- Warm milk and honey
- 1/8–1/4 cup professional/alternative dry food for the evening

Exercise with bag and string.

Heat 1/4–1/2 cup of milk with 1/8 teaspoonful of honey. Make sure it does not boil, that it is lukewarm. Don't forget to leave out his dry food.

T H U R S D A Y

A.M.

- 1/2 can (6 oz.) or one (3 oz.) can kitten food
- 1/8 teaspoon Dr. Jane® Beezyme
- Leave 1/4 cup professional/ alternative dry kitten food just before you leave

Don't forget to pick your kitten up before you leave.

Add more dry food if your kitten was hungry when you got home Wednesday.

comment . . . *Mornings are often very rushed. Take the time to give your kitten a special hug before you leave the house.*

Early P.M.

- Dairy Delight
- Comb/groom
- Exercise
- Antioxidant

RUN AND GET IT
Take that long string with the knot, and let your cat try to catch it, hiding it under the furniture, on the chair, etc. Make that kitten run and get it!

Dairy Delight

1–2 tablespoons of KMR liquid (Pet ag) or milk	1–2 tablespoons of instant rice baby cereal
1 tablespoon cottage cheese	

Mix the instant rice baby cereal with the above ingredients (enough to make the consistency similar to canned kitten food, or a little looser).

DINNER

- 1/2 can (6 oz.) or one (3 oz.) can kitten food
- 1/8 teaspoon Dr. Jane® Beezyme

Remember not to serve cold food.
You should be increasing the amount of Dr. Jane® Beezyme slowly, until you reach 1/8 teaspoon.

comment . . . *Don't forget to feed your kitten in an area that is free from children, adults or any disturbances. Let's give the kitten a chance to develop correct eating habits. We don't want him gobbling his food for fear of disturbance.*

BEFORE BED

- Clean teeth
- 1/4–1/2 cup warm milk and honey
- 1/8–1/4 cup professional/ alternative dry food for the evening

Heat 1/4–1/2 cup of milk with 1/8 teaspoonful of honey.
Make sure it does not boil, that it is lukewarm.
Don't forget to leave out his dry food.

F R I D A Y

A.M.

- 1/2 can (6 oz.) or one (3 oz.) can kitten food
- 1/8 teaspoon Dr. Jane® Beezyme
- Leave 1/4 cup professional/ alternative dry kitten food just before you leave

By now you should be close to the 1/8 teaspoon. If you are not, continue to add a little every day.
By now you should also have an idea of how much food to keep down. You may be down to 1/8 cup, or up to 3/4 cup!

comment . . . By now your kitten is used to the bee pollen and vegetable enzyme (or Dr. Jane® Beezyme). The bee pollen offers nutrients that are not available in kitten food and the vegetable enzyme assures nutrient usage. Neither bee pollen nor vegetable enzyme interferes with food formulation.

Early P.M.

- Veggie–Fruit Bacon Deluxe
- Comb/groom
- Exercise
- Antioxidant

DUNK THE BALL
Dunking the styrofoam ball in the water dish helps acquaint them with water.
Take a deep dish or pot. Fill half with tepid water. Put a styrofoam ball in the water, and watch your kitten play with it.
When it comes time for the kitten's bath you will be glad you played this game!

Veggie—Fruit Bacon Deluxe

Bite-size vegetables, canned or cooked	1–2 pieces cooked bacon
Bite-size fruit, canned or fresh	

Cut up a canned or cooked vegetable into small, bite-size pieces. Also cut up a fruit, canned or fresh, into small bite-size pieces. You can try string beans, peas, lima beans, chopped asparagus. You can try fruits such as canteloupe, avocados, or a vegetable such as corn on the cob (small piece) or nuggets.

Mix together and sprinkle cooked bacon over it.

comment . . . *We are using Fridays to help acquaint your kitten to new food types (fiber) and to water.*

DINNER

- 1/2 can (6 oz.) or one (3 oz.) can kitten food
- 1/8 teaspoon Dr. Jane® Beezyme

Remember not to serve cold food.

BEFORE BED

- Exercise
- Clean teeth
- 1/4–1/2 cup warm milk and honey
- 1/8–1/4 cup dry food for the evening

Any kind of exercise you want.
Heat 1/4–1/2 cup of milk with 1/8 teaspoonful of honey.
Don't forget to leave out his dry food.

comment . . . *If you don't have to go to work Saturday, use this time to get to know your kitten. What type of games does he like? Don't let him play with anything small enough to swallow.*

S A T U R D A Y

A.M.

- Omelet á la Crunch
- Leave 1/4 cup professional/ alternative dry kitten food just before you leave.

Leave dry food for the day as usual.

Omelet á la Crunch

- 1 egg
- 1 tablespoon milk
- Pinch of parsley (fresh is best)
- 1/4 teaspoon chopped raw or cooked vegetables (saved from prior evening)

- Vegetable oil
- 1/4 cup of finely chopped kitten food

Take one egg and beat it. Add a tablespoon of milk, pinch of parsley, and 1/4 teaspoon of chopped raw or cooked vegetable you saved from the prior evening. Put into a frying pan with just enough vegetable oil to coat the pan. Cook the omelet on low. Once it's almost done (the egg is solid), add 1/4 cup of finely chopped kitten food.

Early P.M.

- Yogurt and kitten food
- Comb/groom
- Exercise
- Antioxidant

Select any type of yogurt you want, as long as it has "live culture." Mix 1–3 tablespoons of yogurt with 1/8 cup of kitten food.

Early P.M.

- Exercise
- Antioxidant

CLIMB THE MOUNTAIN
The object of this exercise is to build muscle by climbing. Try to build a multi-level play toy that your cat will climb as it chases that large string with the tie. If you have steps in your house, simply get your kitten to follow you up the stairs by using the string. You can stay on the top, pulling the string slowly toward you. Once the cat reaches the top, send the string back down again—repeating until he has had enough. If you don't have stairs, try a chair with a big, thick back. Trail the string from the seat of the chair to the top, making your cat jump and stretch from the chair seat to the top of the chair.

DINNER

- 1/2 can (6 oz.) or one (3 oz.) can kitten food
- 1/8 teaspoon Dr. Jane® Beezyme

If you are still not at 1/8 teaspoonful, that's okay, but continue to work toward it.

BEFORE BED

- Exercise
- Clean teeth
- Hair-ball medicine
- 1/4–1/2 cup warm milk and honey
- 1/8–1/4 cup dry food for the evening

Use your imagination with your kitten's exercise.

Heat 1/4–1/2 cup of milk with 1/8 teaspoonful of honey. Make sure it does not boil and is lukewarm.

S U N D A Y

A.M.

- 1/2 can (6 oz.) or one (3 oz.) can kitten food
- 1/8 teaspoon Dr. Jane® Beezyme
- 1/4–1/2 cup dry food for the day

Leave dry food for the day as usual.
Don't let your kitten tell you what it will eat.

Early P.M.

- Sunday Afternoon Delight
- Comb/groom
- Clean ears
- Antioxidant

When cleaning the ears: Take a piece of cotton and wet it with ear cleaner from your family veterinarian, or with peroxide mixed with water; 1 part water, 1 part peroxide. Hold your kitten the same as when you brush its teeth. Clean the ears as well as you can, putting your finger into the ear, using the cotton to clean it. *Never use Q-tips!*

Sunday Afternoon Delight

2 tablespoons chopped vegetables (raw or cooked)	1/2 can cat food (3 oz.) or 1/4 can cat food (6 oz.)

Mix the vegetables with the canned cat food.

Weekly examination

Place your kitten on the table as you would to clean its teeth and gums. Mark your rating 1 to 3 in the box below. Go back to the questions for the weekly examination on pages 208–210.

PHYSICAL APPEARANCE	WEEK 1	WEEK 2	WEEK 3	WEEK 4
Looking at your cat from a distance:				
waist line	☐	☐	☐	☐
stomach	☐	☐	☐	☐
Looking at your cat close up:				
whiskers	☐	☐	☐	☐
eyes	☐	☐	☐	☐
breath	☐	☐	☐	☐
coat	☐	☐	☐	☐
skin	☐	☐	☐	☐
tail	☐	☐	☐	☐
nails & pads	☐	☐	☐	☐
ribs	☐	☐	☐	☐
BODILY FUNCTIONS				
appetite	☐	☐	☐	☐
hair balls	☐	☐	☐	☐
stool	☐	☐	☐	☐
BEHAVIOR				
activity	☐	☐	☐	☐

Adult (1 year to 6 years)

Whether your cat is one year old or six, it's probably set in its ways, and they may not be habits that I agree with. Most cats demand dry food at all times, and of course their owners comply. The problem is that most cats begin to gain weight as they increase in age because their metabolism slows down just as ours does. If your cat is not gaining weight, then you can keep dry food down all day; however, if you feel more than a pinch of flesh over the rib cage of your cat, then you have to make a change. If he is just "slightly" overweight, then change to a professional/alternative dry, DIET food. If you really can't find those ribs, then you can't leave dry food down all day. The substitute for the dry food will be vegetables or fruit. Once you find one your cat likes (there are always one or two), then you will slowly increase the substitute and decrease the dry food. You don't have to stop the dry food all at once.

Dry food has its assets, but for the purpose of my 30-day plan, your cat should be eating canned foods. It's impossible to supplement a dry food. Changing from dry to canned food should be done gradually, adding a small amount of canned food (with the supplement) to the dry food, until eventually you are only feeding canned food (the same brand as the dry if possible). Don't worry about any tartar buildup on your cat's teeth because of lack of dry food. Studies are demonstrating that dry food may not help eliminate tooth and gum disease as we once thought.

M O N D A Y

A.M.

- 1/2 can (6 oz.)
OR
- 1 (3 oz.) can adult professional/alternative canned food
- 1/4 teaspoon Dr. Jane® Beezyme
- Leave 1/4–1/2 cup professional/alternative dry adult cat or diet food just before you leave.
- 1/4–1/2 cup chopped vegetables

If you haven't used Dr. Jane® Beezyme before, add just a sprinkle, adding more every meal until you eventually get to 1/4 teaspoon.

Try peas, carrots, asparagus, or string beans. They can be canned, cooked or raw. There is always one vegetable you can find that your cat likes—it's just a matter of trying them.

Use Dr. Jane® Beezyme or equal amounts of bee pollen and vegetable enzyme. If you have not used it before, then just put a slight sprinkle on the food, increasing the amount daily until you arrive at 1/4 teaspoonful. Mix it well.

comment . . . *As cats get older their metabolism tends to get slower, making weight gain easier. Unless your cat is active and does not have a weight problem (lucky him!) you should not leave dry food out all day. Vegetables can be left in place of dry food, giving your cat the fiber he needs without the extra calories. If your cat is in the habit of nibbling on dry food, then it's going to be difficult to change over to vegetables, but it can be done. The best way to change a food habit is to add a tablespoon of chopped vegetables (cooked or raw) into the dry food, adding more vegetables daily, decreasing the amount of dry food until you are serving only vegetables.*

If you can't convert your dry-cat-food nibbler to vegetables, then you must feed him an alternative/professional diet food. Since the dry food represents additional calories, you should not leave more than 1/8–1/4 cup daily. If you have been leaving more than that, start to decrease a little each day. If your cat eats all the dry food immediately after you place it in the bowl, and screams for more during the day, you should serve him small amounts throughout the day until he gets used to dry food control.

Early P.M.

- 1/8 cup dry adult food soaked in 2–4 tablespoons lactose-free milk
- 1/4 teaspoon (or one pump) of Dr. Jane® Feline Formula 1 antioxidants
- Comb/groom
- Exercise
- Liver treats

Don't serve the food cold.

CATNIP IN A SOCK
      Put about 1/4 cup of fresh catnip into a sock. Tie a knot in the sock to keep the catnip from falling out. Take the other end of the sock and let your cat chase after it.

Dr. Jane's Liver Treats

1 cup flour	1/2 cup wheat germ
1 cup cornmeal	1 lb. raw, organic beef or lamb liver
1/4 teaspoon chopped, fresh garlic	1 pinch of salt

Put liver in blender or food processor to liquefy it. (You may want to cut it into small pieces before you blend it.)

Add the above ingredients, mixing well.

Grease a cookie sheet, place 1 large teaspoonful of mixture in rows on the cookie sheet. Flatten the patties with the bottom of a glass dipped in corn meal. Bake at 350° for 15–20 minutes.

CATNIP, not part of the kitten 30-day plan, is added to the adult 30-day plan because catnip is generally liked only by mature cats. It is regarded as an initial stimulant, but then a relaxant. Don't worry when your cat goes ga-ga over the herb—it's harmless and safe.

If your cat has not exercised, start your exercise program slowly. Let him follow the sock for a few minutes, and then give it to him—he will play with it alone.

comment . . . *Depending on the age of your cat, combing, brushing, and exercising may be new to him and may not be well received. Take your time when combing and brushing, rewarding your cat with Dr. Jane's liver treats, or small amount of cat food, and words of praise.*

DINNER

- 1/2 can (6 oz.) or one (3 oz.) can adult food
- 1/4 teaspoon Dr. Jane® Beezyme

The flavor can be different from the morning, however during this 30-day plan, you must keep the same manufacturer you selected for the canned food. The dry food can be from another professional/alternative manufacturer, but that, too, must remain consistent.

If your cat is still not used to the Dr. Jane® Beezyme (or bee pollen), continue to add a small amount, gradually increasing to the 1/4 teaspoon.

BEFORE BED

- Exercise
- Clean teeth
- Hair-ball medicine
- Optional: small-size cooked corn on the cob
- Chopped veggies and fruit
- Optional: lactose-free milk and honey
- 1/8 cup dry adult food or 1/8 cup diet adult food

Catnip sock again (could serve as the reward for brushing the teeth).

Cleaning teeth: If you have not brushed your cat's teeth before, it may not be that simple, but if you can get your cat to accept it, believe me, it's very important.

Hold your cat on a table or counter. Face the head away from you, the tail toward you. Take a toothbrush made for cats, or a finger cot, add toothpaste and put it into your cat's mouth. Lift the gums, and try to brush the back upper teeth, one side at a time. Then try to brush the bottom back teeth, one side at a time. If your cat won't let you do it, stop, and try again tomorrow. Don't forget to reward him.

You can buy any brand of hair-ball medicine from your veterinarian or pet store—different brands have different flavors—the objective is to get a flavor your cat likes! Squeeze it out and let your cat lick it; one good squeeze or pump is enough. If he/she doesn't like it, put it on its nose, or paws—trust me, he will lick it off.

Optional: small-size cooked corn on the cob. Many cats love it—it cleans teeth and gums, just in case you can't! If your cat doesn't like it, that's okay.

Chop 1/4 cup of your cat's favorite cooked or raw vegetable. (You may have to try various types until you find one he/she likes.) Try asparagus, peas, corn nibblets, lima beans, and string beans (raw, canned, or cooked). Fruits include canteloupe, watermelon, berries.

Optional: lactose-free milk and honey (if your cat is not getting fat and is still active at night).

1/8 cup dry or diet, adult food only if your cat is thin or is used to dry food.

1/8 cup diet, adult food if your cat tends to be overweight and is used to dry food.

comment . . . *My goal is to eliminate the dry food at night, replacing it with vegetables. As suggested earlier, try to introduce the veggies and fruits little by little, eventually eliminating the dry food.*

Even though you are leaving down dry food, please leave down the chopped veggies and fruit. Hopefully, your cat will eat that during the night, once the dry food is gone.

T U E S D A Y

A.M.

- 1/2 can (6 oz.) or 1 (3 oz.) can adult professional/ alternative canned food
- 1/4 teaspoon Dr. Jane® Beezyme
- 1/4–1/2 cup chopped veggies
- 1/8–1/4 cup dry food

You can use another flavor, but not a different brand.

If you are still introducing this to your cat, add a little more than you did yesterday—eventually you will get up to 1/4 teaspoon.

Use the dry food only if necessary.

Early P.M.

- 1–2 scrambled eggs
- Exercise
- Antioxidant
- Comb/groom
- Exercise

Scrambled Eggs

1 or 2 eggs	Pinch chopped parsley
Lactose-free milk	Pinch salt

Mix 1 or 2 eggs, depending on your cat's appetite and activity, with just enough lactose-free milk to loosen it. Add a pinch of chopped parsley (fresh is best), and a small pinch of salt. Cook, let it cool and serve.

Use Dr. Jane® Beezyme, but if it is not available use bee pollen and a vegetable enzyme.
Don't forget to reward your cat.

SWING THE STRING
Take a 2–3-inch-wide cord and make it about 6–8 feet long. Tie a big knot at the end. Take that cord and walk or run with it around the house under the furniture, and over—let your cat chase it.

comment . . . If your cat is not used to exercise, or you are not, you better walk with the string—and don't do it for longer than 3–5 minutes. As you and/or your cat get into shape, you can increase the rate of running and the time of play.

DINNER

- 1/2 can (6 oz.) or one (3 oz.) can adult food
- 1/4 teaspoon Dr. Jane® Beezyme

Same brand, but you can vary the flavor.
If you are still adding slowly and haven't gotten to 1/4 teaspoon yet, that's okay. Just increase a little more than you did yesterday and this morning.

BEFORE BED

- Exercise
- Clean teeth
- 1 or 2 soft-boiled eggs
- 1/4–1/2 cup veggies and fruit
- Optional: small-size cooked corn on the cob
- Optional: lactose-free milk and honey

SWING THE STRING
Optional: popcorn. Believe it or not, some cats love it. Just put 1/4 cup into their dish and let them eat it through the night.

- Popcorn
- Dry food if you
  must

comment . . . *This 30-day plan may be very different from what you have been doing. I promise you that once you get into a habit, it will be easy for you, and wait until you see the difference in your cat's health and attitude. If your cat won't eat the veggies that you chose, try different ones tomorrow.*

W E D N E S D A Y

A.M.

- 1/2 can (6 oz.) or 1 (3 oz.) can adult professional/ alternative canned food
- 1/4 teaspoon Dr. Jane® Beezyme
- 1/4–1/2 cup chopped veggies
- Optional: 1/8–1/4 cup dry food

You can use another flavor, but not a different brand.

If you are still introducing the Dr. Jane® Beezyme to your cat, add a little more than you did yesterday—eventually you will get up to 1/4 teaspoon.

Use the dry food only if your cat is still demanding it.

Early P.M.

- Stir-Fry Supreme
- Comb/groom
- Exercise
- Antioxidant

FETCH THE BALL
    Take aluminum foil and make a ball the size of a golf ball. Throw it and let your cat retrieve it. If he won't, then make another 10 balls, throwing them one at a time, to give your cat exercise. You can buy small, foam rubber balls, which are light and fabulous.

Stir-Fry Supreme

1/8 cup chopped, cooked meat or fish	Olive oil
1 tablespoon chopped vegetables	1 tablespoon dry food

Put just enough olive oil in a frying plan to coat the pan, and add the meat or fish and vegetables with one tablespoon of dry food. Mix just long enough to heat and coat everything with the olive oil—DO NOT COOK.

comment . . . *The antioxidant is essential for prevention of disease—especially cancer. Select the one that you prefer.*

DINNER

- 1/2 can (6 oz.) or one (3 oz.) can adult food
- 1/4 teaspoon Dr. Jane® Beezyme

If you still aren't giving this amount of Dr. Jane® Beezyme, it's okay, you will get there.

BEFORE BED

- Exercise
- Clean teeth
- 1/4–1/2 cup veggies and fruit (avocado, canteloupe, watermelon, apple, etc.)
- Optional: lactose-free milk and honey
- Optional: 1/4–1/2 dry adult or diet food

Hopefully you will have gathered all the balls—if not, make more!

You will find a vegetable or fruit your cat likes; it just may take time to get the right one.

Even if your cat doesn't play through the night, and if your cat isn't gaining weight, milk and honey is a great before-bed treat.

comment . . . Some cat owners forget to play with their cats—the cat doesn't often encourage it. It will play by itself or with the other pets in the household. Exercise is vital to your cat's health. It will help keep the heart and muscles strong, and the body in better condition to fight off any type of disease, and it will help keep your cat's figure!

T H U R S D A Y

A.M.

- 1/2 can (6 oz.) or 1 (3 oz.) can food
- 1/4 teaspoon Dr. Jane® Beezyme
- 1/4–1/2 cup chopped veggies
- Optional: 1/8–1/4 cup dry food

You can use another flavor, but not a different brand.

If you are still working up to the 1/4 teaspoon, that's okay—just add a little more today.

If you are still trying to figure out which vegetable your cat likes, that's all right, you will find one. Your cat may not relish veggies as much as dry or canned food, but you know best for him.

Use the dry food only if your cat is still demanding it.

comment . . . *You may need to vary the amount of food you are feeding, depending on your cat's metabolism. On Sunday you will evaluate your cat's weight, and determine if you need to decrease or increase the amount of food you are feeding.*

Early P.M.

- Yogurt delight
- Comb/groom
- Exercise
- Antioxidant

1/4 cup plain yogurt (with live culture). Mix it with 2 tablespoons of dry food.

JUMP AND CATCH
You can buy a "kitty tease" or an actual fishing pole on which you would tie a catnip toy. Some people use a broom handle. The object is to let the pole do the work for you! Let your cat try to catch the prey!

DINNER

- 1/2 can (6 oz.) or one (3 oz.) can adult food
- 1/4 teaspoon Dr. Jane® Beezyme

If you still aren't giving this amount of Dr. Jane® Beezyme, it's okay—you will get there.

BEFORE BED

- Exercise
- Clean teeth
- 1/4–1/2 cup veggies and fruit
- Optional: lactose-free milk and honey
- Optional: 1/4–1/2 dry adult or diet food

JUMP AND CATCH

comment . . . *Every cat is different, as is every cat owner, so I have made these daily schedules as simple as I could. The grooming, playing, and preparing of meals will increase the bond between you and your cat. You will notice things about him that you never did before. That's important—he can't talk to you, so you have to do your best to understand his needs. My 30-day plan is designed to fullfill these needs.*

F R I D A Y

A.M.

- 1/2 can (6 oz.) or 1 (3 oz.) can food
- 1/4 teaspoon Dr. Jane® Beezyme
- 1/4–1/2 cup chopped veggies
- Optional: 1/8–1/4 cup dry food

If you are still increasing the Dr. Jane® Beezyme, that's okay—just add a little more today.

Early P.M.

- Fish for Friday
- Comb/groom
- Exercise
- Antioxidant

DUNK THE STYROFOAM BALL
    Take a spaghetti pot and fill it half way with tepid water. Take the foam ball you play with, or get a styrofoam ball—see if you can get your cat to play with it. This exercise is more mental than physical.

Fish for Friday

2 oz. white-meat fish with no bones (cod, fillet of sole)	Pinch of salt
1/4 cup cooked, brown rice	1/4 clove chopped garlic
1/4 teaspoon olive oil	pinch of crushed parsley, fresh parsley is the best
1/2 teaspoon butter	1/8 teaspoon Dr. Jane® Beezyme

Sauté garlic in the oil and butter. Add fish until cooked. Then add the rice and mix well, mashing the rice with a fork. Add salt, Beezyme and parsley. Put into a dish and serve when cool.

comment . . . *If the recipe and/or the above exercise is too much for you, you can substitute it for any of the other afternoon exercises and recipes.*

DINNER

- 1/2 can (6 oz.) or one (3 oz.) can adult food
- 1/4 teaspoon Dr. Jane® Beezyme

If you still aren't giving this amount of Dr. Jane® Beezyme, it's okay.

BEFORE BED

- Exercise
- Clean teeth
- 1/4–1/2 cup veggies and fruit
- Optional: lactose-free milk and honey
- Optional: corn on the cob
- Optional: popcorn
- Optional: 1/4–1/2 cup dry adult or diet food

You pick the exercise tonight.

comment . . . *Friday is often the last day of work, which means that you can spend more time with your cat. This is the perfect time to try new vegetables and fruits.*

S A T U R D A Y

A.M.

Eggs and Bacon á la Crunch

Eggs and Bacon á la Crunch

| 1 soft-boiled egg | 1/8 cup dry food, optional |
| 1 piece bacon minced | |

Mix the dry food with the egg and minced bacon. Let it cool and serve.

Early P.M.

- Liver Deluxe
- Comb/groom
- Exercise
- Antioxidant

CLIMB THE MOUNTAIN

The object of this exercise is to maintain muscle and burn calories by climbing. Try to buy or build a multi-level play toy (Tree House Original's have natural bark tree houses of all types). Take the large string with the knot at the end, and get your cat to follow it up the tree house, or up over the couch, up onto the counter, chair, etc. Take it easy if your cat is not used to this physical activity. You can start with one minute and work your way up to fifteen!

Liver Deluxe

1–2 livers, chopped	1/4 teaspoon olive oil
1/4 clove garlic, chopped	Pinch of salt
1 teaspoon butter	

Sauté the garlic in a frying pan with butter and oil. Add the chicken and cook until done. Let it cool and serve.

comment... *Try to keep the pieces large so that it helps clean the teeth and gums! Liver supplies vital nutritional components.*

DINNER

- 1/2 can (6 oz.) or one (3 oz.) can adult food
- 1/4 teaspoon Dr. Jane® Beezyme

If you still aren't giving this amount of Dr. Jane® Beezyme, it's okay, you will get there.

BEFORE BED

- Exercise
- Clean teeth
- Hair-ball medicine
- 1/4–1/2 cup veggies and fruit
- Optional: corn on the cob
- Optional: 1/4–1/2 cup dry adult or diet food

If your cat has long hair you may want to give hair-ball medicine again on Sunday.

S U N D A Y

A.M.

- 1/2 can (6 oz.) or 1 (3 oz.) can food
- 1/2 teaspoon Dr. Jane® Beezyme
- 1/4–1/2 cup veggies
- Optional: 1/4–1/2 cup adult or diet dry food

If you still aren't giving this amount of Dr. Jane® Beezyme, it's okay—you will get there. It's very important to provide your cat with nutrients not found in most commercial pet foods.

Early P.M.

- Stir-Fry Supreme
- Comb/groom
- Exercise
- Antioxidant

Stir-Fry Supreme

1/8 cup chopped, cooked meat or fish	olive oil
1 tablespoon chopped vegetables	1 tablespoon dry food

Put just enough olive oil in a frying pan to coat the pan. Add the meat or fish and vegetables with one tablespoon of dry food. Mix just long enough to heat and coat everything with the olive oil—DO NOT COOK.

Exercise can be anything you want—you can even rest for this afternoon!

DINNER

- 1/2 can (6 oz.) or one (3 oz.) can adult food
- 1/4 teaspoon Dr. Jane® Beezyme

You should give 1/4 teaspoon of Dr. Jane® Beezyme, or at least close to it by now.

BEFORE BED

- Exercise
- Clean teeth
- 1/4–1/2 cup veggies and fruit
- Optional: lactose-free milk and honey
- Optional: corn on the cob
- Optional: 1/4–1/2 cup dry adult or diet food
- Make sure kitty greens are available

KITTY GREENS: This is the healthiest, natural way for your cat to get his plant nutrients. If you have never grown kitty greens before, don't worry, you don't need a green thumb.

Cleaning Ears: Take a piece of cotton and wet it with ear cleaner from your family veterinarian, or with peroxide mixed with water; 1 part water, 1 part peroxide. Clean the ears as well as you can, putting your finger into the ear, using the cotton to clean it. Never use Q-tips!

comment . . . *The next week will be a lot easier with a well-developed routine. If you are not giving the full amount of supplement, that's okay, just continue to introduce a little at a time until you reach the suggested amount.*

The most important parts of this weekly plan are the exercise, antioxidant and the bee pollen plus vegetable enzyme (Dr. Jane® Beezyme). Exercise is vital to your cat's health. Once you start an exercise program with which both you and your cat agree, it will become a part of your routine.

Weekly examination

Place your cat on the table as you would to clean its teeth and gums. Mark your rating 1 to 3 in the box below. Go back to the questions for the weekly examination on pages 208–210.

PHYSICAL APPEARANCE	WEEK 1	WEEK 2	WEEK 3	WEEK 4
Looking at your cat from a distance:				
waist line	☐	☐	☐	☐
stomach	☐	☐	☐	☐
Looking at your cat close up:				
whiskers	☐	☐	☐	☐
eyes	☐	☐	☐	☐
breath	☐	☐	☐	☐
coat	☐	☐	☐	☐
skin	☐	☐	☐	☐
tail	☐	☐	☐	☐
nails & pads	☐	☐	☐	☐
ribs	☐	☐	☐	☐
BODILY FUNCTIONS				
appetite	☐	☐	☐	☐
hair balls	☐	☐	☐	☐
stool	☐	☐	☐	☐
BEHAVIOR				
activity	☐	☐	☐	☐

Geriatric (Cat 6 Years +)

Older cats have special needs depending on the condition of their health—even if they don't appear to be sick, prevention is critical if we want them to live long and happy lives. The aging process affects the entire body, decreasing the efficiency of the body to function. We may not see the very slight daily changes, but every body process is involved. We see the degeneration once the body is no longer able to compensate, and we see the "disease" state. Cataract formation, kidney disease and heart disease, constipation, arthritis, and cancer are just a few of the common maladies seen in older cats.

This diet plan is designed for the "healthy" older cat and does not include intervention for specific disease. No matter what age your geriatric cat is, if you follow my 30-day plan you will see a remarkable difference in your cat's quality of life and very importantly, you will delay the negative effects of aging.

As we all know, the cat is a creature of habit and it is difficult to make changes in its life. It is essential that your cat eat canned food for this 30-day regimen to be successful. The geriatric supplement has to be added; it's impossible to add the supplement to dry food. If your cat does not eat canned food, add a small amount of professional/alternative canned food to the dry food. If you are already feeding a professional/alternative dry food, then add the SAME manufacturer's canned food, not another brand. Add a small amount of the geriatric supplement to that small amount of canned food, slowly increasing the amount of canned food and a geriatric supplement. Your goal is to convert your cat from dry to canned food within a few weeks. If you can't get your cat to change altogether, but are successful in adding the entire amount of geriatric supplement into the amount of canned food that you are adding to the dry food, that's okay.

You have to be willful regarding one more item; leaving dry food down all day. If you have been doing this, and your cat is overweight, you have to make a change. The dry food must be a professional/ alternative DIET food that you will gradually substitute with vegetables and/or fruit. You will simply try various types of vegetables and fruits until you find one that your cat will accept. Then you add a small amount of the vegetable or fruit to the dry food, reducing the amount of dry food slowly, until your cat no longer wants dry food. Again, take a few weeks for this change, but be sure to make it!

M O N D A Y

A.M.

- 1/2 can (6 oz.) or 1 (3 oz.) can adult professional/alternative canned food

OR

- 1/4 cup dry diet professional/alternative food with 1 teaspoon professional/alternative canned food
- Pinch of the Geriatric Supplement Mixture + 1/8 teaspoon of water
- 1/4 cup chopped vegetables (lima beans, string beans, corn nuggets, peas, no sugar)
- Optional: 1/8 cup professional/alternative dry cat food (diet or adult)

If your cat does not eat canned food, feed it almost 1/4 cup professional/alternative food with 1 teaspoon of canned. We have to be able to add the Geriatric Supplement Mixture.

Leave out the vegetables in place of the dry food.

Geriatric Supplement Mixture

1/4 teaspoon bee pollen	1/4 teaspoon Dr. Jane® Beezyme
1/8 teaspoon oat bran	1/8 teaspoon oat bran
1/8 teaspoon fresh garlic (from jar or minced) **OR**	1/8 teaspoon fresh garlic (from jar or minced)
1/4 teaspoon of Prozyme® *	

Combine the above ingredients and add to food.

comment . . . You can make one week's worth of this mixture on Sunday night, so that all you have to do is add 1/8 teaspoon of the mixture daily, rather than combining them separately.

WEEKLY GERIATRIC SUPPLEMENT MIXTURE:

1 3/4 teaspoons bee pollen
1 teaspoon oat bran
1 teaspoon fresh garlic (jar or minced)
1 3/4 teaspoons Prozyme®

OR

1 3/4 teaspoons Dr. Jane® Beezyme
1 teaspoon oat bran
1 teaspoon fresh garlic (from jar or minced)

comment . . . Since your cat has never had these supplements before, just add a sprinkle of the GERIATRIC SUPPLEMENT MIXTURE, increasing the amount daily until you are able to give the indicated amounts.

* **Prozyme** is a brand of natural vegetable enzymes. This remarkable formula, studied at the Mayo Clinic Laboratories, increases the digestion of nutrients. If you can't get the Prozyme, there are other vegetable enzymes.

* **Dr. Jane® Beezyme** is my formulation, which includes enzymes and bee pollen. If you can't get it, then mix bee pollen with a vegetable enzyme.

Early P.M.

- 1/2 teaspoon of canned food
- 3–5 nuggets of dry food
- Sprinkle of water
- Comb/groom
- Exercise
- Antioxidant

Add just enough water to allow the dry food to soften. Combine it with the canned food.

The Dr. Jane® Feline Formula One was designed to be easy to give (it's a gel that your cat licks off if you put it on its nose or paws). If you can't find this formula, select another antioxidant formula.

Comb and Groom: Make sure that your brush is appropriate—not too soft and not too hard. Place your cat on a table, with the head away from you, tail toward you. Brush backward, from tail to head, and then head to tail. During flea season, follow with a flea comb, combing from head to tail. Remove the dead hair and flea dirt into the toilet.

ISOMETRIC STRETCH

Using a kitty tease, or a long pole with a feather or bow tied on it, let your cat try to reach for it. Depending on the age and agility of your cat, you can make your cat really stretch, and if young enough, jump for it.

DINNER

- 1 (3 oz.) can or 1/2 (6 oz.) can of canned food
- 1/4 teaspoon canned pumpkin or 1/4 teaspoon instant oatmeal
- 1/4 teaspoon Beezyme®

Since your cat has not had pumpkin or oatmeal before, you may have to add less than the amount required, working your way up, day by day.

Take the pumpkin from the can and put into ice-cube trays. Use one cube per 1–2 days, letting it defrost in the refrigerator in a plastic bag.

Use Dr. Jane® Beezyme, but if it is not available, mix equal parts bee pollen with a vegetable enzyme.

BEFORE BED

- Exercise
- Clean teeth
- Hair-ball medicine
- 1/4 cup chopped vegetables
- Corn on the cob
- Optional: 1/3 cup dry adult or diet food

ISOMETRIC STRETCH

Cleaning teeth: Hold your cat on a table or counter. Face its head away from you, the tail towards you. Take a toothbrush made for cats, or a finger cot, add toothpaste and put it into your cat's mouth. Lift the lips, and try to brush the back upper teeth, one side at a time. Then try to brush the bottom back teeth, one side at a time. If your cat won't let you do it—stop, and try again tomorrow. Don't forget to reward him.

Give one pump or squeeze of hair-ball medicine. There are many types on the market; they vary in flavor.

Corn on the cob. Some cats love it and it's great for teeth and gums, even though it's a little messy.

If your cat didn't like the vegetables you chose during the morning, let's try another one.

Leave the dry food, only if your cat is used to it and insists. Remember, the goal is to substitute vegetables for dry food.

comment . . . *All of this may seem like a lot, but once you get into the routine, it is very simple. The hardest part of this is introducing your cat to vegetables. Do what you can—if you can't follow this plan 100%, that's okay.*

T U E S D A Y

A.M.

- 1/2 (6 oz.) or 1 (3 oz.) can professional/ alternative food
- 1/8 teaspoon geriatric supplement
- 1/4 cup chopped veggies
- Optional: 1/4–1/2 cup adult or diet dry food

You may change the flavor, but you must not change the brand of canned food you have selected.

You will probably add only 2 pinches, still working your way up to the 1/8 teaspoon supplement.

Leave the vegtables out throughout the day.

You must use the same dry food throughout the 30-day diet plan.

Early P.M.

- 1/2 teaspoon canned food
- 3–5 nuggets of dry food
- Comb/groom
- Exercise
- Antioxidant

Add just enough water to allow the dry food to soften, and add the canned food.

SWING THE STRING

Take a 3-inch-wide string and cut it to about 6 or 8 ft. Tie a knot on the end. Walk around the house with the string, letting your cat follow it. If you don't want to walk, simply toss it to various places, pulling it toward you while your cat follows. Do this for a minimum of 5 minutes if your cat is in good health; otherwise use your judgment.

DINNER

- 1 (3 oz.) can food or 1/2 (6 oz.) can food
- 1/4 teaspoon canned pumpkin or 1/4 teaspoon instant oatmeal
- 1/4 teaspoon Dr. Jane® Beezyme

You should still be increasing the pumpkin until you reach 1/4 teaspoon.

comment . . . You are probably not adding the 1/4 teaspoon of fiber and Dr. Jane® Beezyme yet. That's okay, just be sure to increase it little by little so that you can get up to that amount. If your cat has refused his dinner, you probably added too much of the supplements.

BEFORE BED

- Exercise
- Clean teeth
- 1/4 cup chopped veggies
- Corn on the cob
- Optional: popcorn
- Optional: 1/3 cup dry adult or diet food

SWING THE STRING

You may have to still try a new vegetable. If you've found one your cat likes, that's great.

Yes, some cats love the crunch of popcorn and that can be the replacement for dry food if your cat refuses all the vegetables that you select.

Dry food if necessary.

W E D N E S D A Y

A.M.

- 1/2 (6 oz.) or 1 (3 oz.) can professional/alternative food
- 1/8 teaspoon geriatric supplement
- 1/4 cup chopped veggies
- Optional: 1/4–1/2 cup adult or diet dry food

Even if your cat just nibbled on the vegetables you selected, that's a beginning, and use that same vegetable again. If not, select another one.

comment . . . *By this time you can see that this plan is not as difficult as you thought. Wait until you see how great your cat looks within a few weeks!*

Early P.M.

- 1 soft-boiled egg + 3–5 nuggets dry food
- Comb/groom
- Exercise
- Antioxidant

The dry food can be crushed if your cat is not used to it or can't chew it.

FOLLOW THE CATNIP SOCK

Take 4 tablespoons of catnip and put it into a sock. Tie the sock. Then take the catnip sock and move it around, up on the couch, around the floor, etc. Only do the amount of exercise your cat is used to. Again, 5 minutes is the minimum (unless he has any difficulty). These exercises are crucial to his better health.

DINNER

- 1 (3 oz.) can food or 1/2 (6 oz.) can food
- 1/4 teaspoon canned pumpkin or 1/4 teaspoon instant oatmeal
- 1/4 teaspoon Dr. Jane® Beezyme

You should still be increasing the pumpkin until you reach 1/4 teaspoon.

BEFORE BED

- Exercise
- Clean teeth
- 1/2 cup warm lactose-free milk + 1/8 teaspoon honey
- 1/3 cup canteloupe or avocado or watermelon
- Optional: 1/3 cup dry adult or diet food.

FOLLOW THE CATNIP SOCK

Heat the milk—don't bring it to a boil. Add the honey, and let the milk cool to room temperature before you give it to your cat.

If your cat refuses fruits, it's okay. Fruit is just another option in case we can't get him to eat vegetables.

T H U R S D A Y

A.M.

- 1/2 (6 oz.) or 1 (3 oz.) can professional/alternative food
- 1/8 teaspoon geriatric supplement
- 1/4 cup chopped veggies
- Optional: 1/4–1/2 cup adult or diet dry food

While it's preferable not to leave food out all day, if your cat is not gaining weight from the dry food, you can leave it for him to nibble on all day. I still want vegetables added to the diet so be sure to leave them out throughout the day, in a separate dish.

Early P.M.

- Scrambled eggs & Parsley
- Comb/groom
- Exercise
- Antioxidant

Scrambled Eggs & Parsley

1–2 eggs
1/2 teaspoon lactose-free milk

Pinch of parsley (fresh is best)

Mix eggs with 1/2 teaspoon lactose-free milk with a pinch of parsley. Cook until done. Let it cool and serve with a pinch of salt.

DINNER

- 1/2 (6 oz.) can food or 1 (3 oz.) can food
- 1/4 teaspoon canned pumpkin or 1/4 teaspoon instant oatmeal
- 1/4 teaspoon Dr. Jane® Beezyme

BEFORE BED

- Exercise
- Clean teeth
- 1/3 cup corn nuggets
- Optional: 1/3 cup dry adult or diet food

FISHING WE GO
    Use a kitty tease or make a fishing pole from a broomstick, or buy an actual, inexpensive fishing pole. Tie a catnip sock, string, or some type of feather on the end. Let your cat chase it—at his speed.

F   R   I   D   A   Y

A.M.

- 1/2 (6 oz.) or 1 (3 oz.) can professional/ alternative food
- 1/8 teaspoon geriatric supplement
- 1/3 cup corn nuggets
- Optional: 1/3 cup adult or diet dry food

Don't forget that you can change the flavor, not the brand.
    If your cat does not eat canned food, then add a small amount of professional/alternative canned food to the dry food. If you are already feeding a professional/alternative dry food, then add the SAME brand canned food, not another brand. Your goal is to convert your cat from dry to canned food within a few weeks.
    Put the corn nuggets in a separate dish.

Early P.M.

- Fish Fillet & Garlic
- Comb/groom
- Exercise
- Antioxidant

Fish Fillet & Garlic

- White-meat fish (cod, sole)
- 1/8 teaspoon garlic
- Olive oil
- Sprinkle of parsley
- Pinch of salt

Sauté 1/8 teaspoon garlic in enough olive oil to moisten the frying pan. Cook the "white-meat fish" (cod, sole), making sure there are no bones. Sprinkle parsley (fresh is best), add a pinch of salt and serve.

comment . . . *The antioxidant is essential to your cat's health. Choose the form that's best for you and your cat: powder, water or paste.*

STRING AND BAG
Take that long string and place it in a paper bag. Let your cat pounce on it and stalk it. Repeat for 5 minutes or until your cat gets tired.

DINNER

- 1 (3 oz.) can food or 1/2 (6 oz.) can food
- 1/4 teaspoon canned pumpkin or 1/4 teaspoon instant oatmeal
- 1/4 teaspoon Dr. Jane® Beezyme

You may think that the dinners are redundant, and you are right. We have to get your older cat into the habit of eating what is healthy.

BEFORE BED

- Exercise
- Clean teeth
- 1 squeeze of hairball medicine
- 1/4 cup veggies
- Optional: 1/3 cup dry adult or diet food

You can do any kind of exercise you want with your cat. Have fun!

S A T U R D A Y

A.M.

- 1/2 (6 oz.) or 1 (3 oz.) can professional/ alternative food
- 1/8 teaspoon geriatric supplement
- 1/4 cup veggies
- Optional: 1/3 cup adult or diet dry food

If you still have not succeeded in getting your cat to eat a vegetable, this is the time to try another one. Take the time to offer it raw and if that doesn't work, cook it.

Leave the vegetables out during the day as a substitute for dry food.

Early P.M.

- Liver Delight
- Comb/Groom
- Exercise
- Antioxidant

Liver Delight

1/2 cup diced liver	1/8 teaspoon minced vegetables
1/8 teaspoon minced garlic	

Combine liver, garlic and vegetables. Sauté all of it in a small amount of olive oil until done. Let it cool and serve.

FETCH THE BALL

Take aluminum foil and make it into a ball about the size of a small golf ball, or buy small, foam rubber golf balls. These are so light that when you throw them your cat may retrieve them. If not, that's okay. Just make sure you have at least 4 to throw, so your cat goes after it four times. If he stops at two that's okay.

DINNER

- 1 (3 oz.) can food or 1/2 (6 oz.) can food
- 1/8 teaspoon geriatric supplement

You should be up to 1/8 teaspoon of the geriatric supplement; if not, keep trying.

BEFORE BED

- Clean teeth
- Hair-ball medicine
- 1/4 cup veggies
- Optional: corn on the cob
- Optional: popcorn
- Optional: 1/3 cup dry adult or diet food

No exercises tonight. Relax.
Let's not forget 1 squeeze of the hair-ball medicine.

comment . . . *By this time, your cat is getting used to eating healthy. Use Saturday to work on the parts of this plan that are not going smooth (i.e., brushing your cat's teeth). Perhaps you should take a different approach, such as holding him on your lap, with head away from you and tail towards you. Use a finger cot rather than a brush, and perhaps you should try a different flavor toothpaste.*

I can't over-emphasize exercise. If you or your cat don't like the ones I have given you, do others. The point is to exercise, but gradually build up exercise routines if your cat is not used to it.

If you haven't grown wheat grass in a small flower pot for your cat to nibble on, today may be a great day to do so. Just get seeds, potting soil, a pot and plant the seeds. Don't forget to water them. Leave them in a partially sunny room. It's the best fiber and nutrient source money can buy!

S U N D A Y

A.M.

- 1/2 (6 oz.) or 1 (3 oz.) can food
- 1/8 teaspoon geriatric supplement
- 1/3 cup veggies
- Optional: 1/3 cup adult or diet dry food

Early P.M.

- Fat-Free Cottage Cheese á la Crunch
- Comb/groom
- Exercise
- Antioxidant

CLIMB THE MOUNTAIN
The object of this exercise is to build muscle by climbing. Set up your furniture so that your cat has to walk or jump from one level to another, or using that long cord, get your cat to go up and down stairs (you can go along for the exercise, too). You may want to have your cat go from the floor, to a foot bench, to the couch, to the top of the couch, and then back down.

Fat-Free Cottage Cheese á la Crunch

1–3 tablespoons cottage cheese	3–5 nuggets dry food, minced

Mix cottage cheese with dry, minced nuggets. Mix very well and serve.

If your cat does not like dry food, then save one teaspoon of food from the morning and add that to the cottage cheese.

BEFORE BED

- Clean teeth
- Clean ears
- 1/3 cup corn nuggets or baby peas (without sugar)
- Optional: 1/3 cup dry adult or diet food

If you find that your cat is getting fat, cut down on the dry food and decrease the amount of canned food by 1/3.

comment . . . *The next week will be a lot easier since you will have developed a routine. Try to reach the amounts of supplement that I recommend by the end of the second week. If you can't, that's okay—do what you can.*

The most important part of this plan is breakfast and dinner with the GERIATRIC SUPPLEMENT MIXTURE. Exercise is the second most important part of the plan, with the vegetables and fruit and snacks important, but not essential. The afternoon snacks are designed to deliver certain additional nutrients to your cat's diet. If you can't make them, or your cat just doesn't eat them, that's okay—do the best you can. The better your cat looks and acts, the more encouraged you will be.

Don't forget that every brushing and combing comes with TLC. All cats need that—it's an essential component of this 30-day plan.

Weekly examination

Place your cat on the table as you would to clean its teeth and gums. Mark your rating 1 to 3 in the box below. Go back to the questions for the weekly examination on pages 208–210.

	WEEK 1	WEEK 2	WEEK 3	WEEK 4
PHYSICAL APPEARANCE Looking at your cat from a distance:				
waist line	☐	☐	☐	☐
stomach	☐	☐	☐	☐
Looking at your cat close up:				
whiskers	☐	☐	☐	☐
eyes	☐	☐	☐	☐
breath	☐	☐	☐	☐
coat	☐	☐	☐	☐
skin	☐	☐	☐	☐
tail	☐	☐	☐	☐
nails & pads	☐	☐	☐	☐
ribs	☐	☐	☐	☐
BODILY FUNCTIONS				
appetite	☐	☐	☐	☐
hairballs	☐	☐	☐	☐
stool	☐	☐	☐	☐
BEHAVIOR				
activity	☐	☐	☐	☐

Obese Cat

Cats, just like us, start to gain weight and we don't even realize it. To determine if your cat is overweight, you need to do the feel test on page 175. If there is more than one inch of fat, then you want to follow this 30-day regime.

Please don't take obesity lightly (see page 280). This diet plan is designed for the "healthy OVERWEIGHT cat" and does not include intervention for specific disease. No matter what age your overweight cat is, if you follow my 30-day plan you will see a remarkable difference in your cat's quality of life and, very importantly, you will be delaying the negative effects of excess weight.

If your cat is used to eating dry food, all day long, it must eat a professional/alternative DIET dry food, and that's only until you have converted him to vegetables or fruits. There is always a vegetable or fruit that a cat will eat, it's just a matter of trying different types, cooked or fresh, until your cat agrees to eat one, even if it's not with the voraciousness that it eats the dry food. Once you have found that fruit or vegetable, then you have to mix it with the dry food, decreasing the dry food daily, until your cat is eating only the vegetable or fruit, forgetting about the dry food forever.

If your cat will eat ONLY dry food, then you have to introduce it to canned food in order to add supplements. Again, select a canned professional/alternative diet food (the same brand as the dry, if possible), and add a small amount of canned food to the dry food, mixing well. Day by day, you will add more canned, and feed less dry food, until you can get all of the supplement into the canned food and into your cat. If you end up mixing canned and dry, that's okay, as long as they are both professional/alternative and have the amount of supplements I suggest.

M O N D A Y

A.M.

- 1/2 can professional/alternative canned diet food

OR

- 1/2 cup dry diet professional/alternative food with 1 teaspoon professional/alternative canned food
- 1 pinch of SLIM & HEALTHY SUPPLE-MENT MIXTURE
- 1/4 cup chopped vegetables (peas, string beans, asparagus, lima beans)
- Optional: 1/3 cup dry professional/alternative diet food

The dosage of the SLIM & HEALTHY SUPPLEMENT should be 1/8 teaspoon, but since it's something different, cats will usually only tolerate new things when they are offered in small amounts—a pinch is a great way to start!

Leave the vegetables out, in a separate dish, during the day.

Slim & Healthy Supplement Mixture

1/4 teaspoon Dr. Jane® Beezyme	If you can't find Dr. Jane® Beezyme, then substitute with:
1/8 teaspoon minced, fresh parsley	
	1/8 teaspoon bee pollen
1/8 teaspoon minced rosemary	1/8 teaspoon Prozyme®*

Mix all the ingredients together and sprinkle on food as directed.

* **Prozyme®** is a brand of natural vegetable enzymes. This remarkable formula, as shown by studies at the Mayo Clinic Laboratories, increases the digestion of nutrients. If you can't get the Prozyme, use a vegetable enzyme.

comment . . . *You can mix up one batch of Slim & Healthy Supplement Mixture weekly; keep it in a jar (no plastic) and use as directed.*

Early P.M.

- 1/4 can food with a pinch of fresh or powdered dandelion or 3 drops of tincture

OR

- 1/4 cup dry food and 1 teaspoon canned food with a pinch of fresh or powdered dandelion or 2 drops of tincture.
- Comb/groom
- Exercise
- Antioxidant

Use Dr. Jane® Beezyme, but if it is not available, use bee pollen and a vegetable enzyme.

Comb/groom: Many heavy cats have difficulty grooming themselves, so this is a great opportunity to help them. Pay particular attention to the back end, around the tail, especially if he is a long-haired cat. Never lift up the tail, gently hold it up, taking a look and then trying to comb or brush the tail. Your cat should be on a table or counter facing away from you, tail toward you, with no restraint, just TLC. If you find matted hair under the tail, try to comb it gently; if you don't succeed today, you can try again tomorrow. If you can't get out the mats, then you will have to bring your cat to a groomer or veterinarian. Mats attract dirt, insects, and they are uncomfortable.

WALK THE STRING

Take a 3-inch-wide cord and cut to 6- or 8-ft. length. Tie a knot at the end. Walk around with the string and let your cat follow. At least 5 minutes is necessary. Go slow, if he is not used to exercise; otherwise, go fast. If you don't want to walk around, cast the string over the couch, around the chair, etc., pulling it toward you, while your cat tries to catch it. The more strenuous, the more calories burned, but if your cat is not conditioned, go slowly!

comment . . . *Non-alcoholic dandelion tincture can be purchased from Animals' Apawthecary (1-800-822-9609).*

DINNER

- 1/4 can professional/alternative diet food

OR

- Just a little less than 1/4 cup dry professional/alternative food with 1 teaspoon professional/alternative canned food
- 1 pinch of SLIM & HEALTHY SUPPLEMENT MIXTURE
- 1/4 cup chopped vegetables (peas, string beans, asparagus, lima beans)
- Optional: 1/3 cup dry professional/alternative diet food

You can change flavors, but make sure that you stay with the brand of canned food selected.

If you are also leaving down dry food, reduce the amount of food (dry or canned) by about 10%.

If your cat tolerated the morning dose of the supplement mixture, let's go up to two pinches—our ultimate goal is 1/8 teaspoon.

Leave the vegetables out, in a separate dish, during the day.

BEFORE BED

- Exercise
- Clean teeth
- hair-ball medicine
- 1/4 cup veggies
- Optional: corn on the cob
- Optional: popcorn
- Optional: 1/3 cup dry adult or diet food

WALK THE STRING

Cleaning Teeth: Place your cat on a counter or table, with his head away from you just as you did for grooming. Take a cat toothbrush or finger cot and put feline toothpaste on it. Slowly lift up your cat's upper lip and rub the back teeth. Then do the other side. If your cat rebels, that's to be expected; you will try again tomorrow.

There are many types of hair-ball medicine on the market, each with their own flavor. You have to select the one your cat likes best.

Many cats love cooked corn on the cob. It's not fattening and helps clean teeth and gums.

If the vegetables you selected this morning were not appealing to your cat, try another one tonight. Don't despair, you will find one.

comment . . . *This 30-day plan is not just about weight loss. It's about general health, and that's why I have included brushing teeth and general grooming. The additional time you are spending with your cat, taking care of him, will also enhance your relationship.*

T U E S D A Y

A.M.

- 1/2 can professional/ alternative diet food

OR

- Just a little less than 1/2 cup dry diet professional/ alternative food with 1 teaspoon professional/ alternative canned food
- 1/8 teaspoon SLIM & HEALTHY SUPPLEMENT MIXTURE
- 1/4 cup chopped veggies
- Optional: 1/3 cup dry professional/ alternative diet food

You are probably not able to put in 1/8 teaspoon of the Slim & Healthy Supplement Mixture yet, so add 1–2 pinches; you will work up to the 1/8 teaspoon by the end of the week or early the next week.

If your cat didn't like the vegetables you offered him yesterday, try offering the same ones, either raw or cooked; sometimes it's just a matter of "mouth feel."

Leave the vegetables out, in a separate dish, during the day.

Early P.M.

- 1/4 can food with a pinch of fresh or powdered dande- lion or 2 drops of tincture

OR

- 1/4 cup dry food + 1 teaspoon canned food with a pinch of fresh or pow- dered dandelion or 2 drops of tincture
- Comb/groom
- Exercise
- Antioxidant

You may not be able to add that much of the herb today; it may take time to get your cat used to this amount. Make a real effort because it will help your cat lose weight and it's really a healthy supplement.

ISOMETRIC STRETCH AND CATCH

Take a fishing pole, or a broomstick, and tie onto it a catnip sock, or a feather or something that your cat will want to chase. Hold it above his head and let's see a big stretch, and then let your cat chase it. Again, a minimum of five minutes is required to burn some calories, but if your cat can just stretch, that's okay.

comment . . . *The more often a cat eats, the more calories he burns, however, even though he eats more frequently, you must be careful not to give him MORE food than you normally would.*

DINNER
- 1/4 can professional/alternative diet food

OR
- Just a little less than 1/4 cup dry professional/alternative food with 1 teaspoon professional/alternative canned food
- 1/8 teaspoon SLIM & HEALTHY SUPPLEMENT MIXTURE

BEFORE BED
- Exercise
- Clean teeth
- Hair-ball medicine
- 1/4 cup corn nuggets
- Optional: corn on the cob
- Optional: popcorn
- Optional: 1/3 cup dry adult or diet food

ISOMETRIC STRETCH AND CATCH

If you are leaving down dry food for nibbling during the night, don't forget to cut down by 25% the amount of dinner you are feeding.

W E D N E S D A Y

A.M.
- 1/2 can professional/ alternative diet food

OR
- Just a little less than 1/2 cup dry diet professional/ alternative food with 1 teaspoon professional/ alternative canned food
- 1/8 teaspoon SLIM & HEALTHY SUPPLEMENT MIXTURE
- 1/4 cup chopped vegetables
- Optional: 1/3 cup dry professional/ alternative diet food

Don't forget to keep the same brand of dry professional/alternative food as you have been feeding.

Leave the vegetables out, in a separate dish, during the day.

Early P.M.

- 1 soft-boiled egg + 3–5 nuggets dry food
- a pinch of dandelions (fresh if possible) or 2 drops of non-alcoholic dandelion tincture
- Comb/groom
- Exercise
- Antioxidant

You may not be able to add that much of the herb today; it may take time to get your cat used to this amount.

STRING AND BAG

Take that 3-inch cord with the knot and hide the knot in a paper bag. Let your cat chase it, and chase it, for at least five minutes. If he can't, don't continue the exercise.

comment . . . *Antioxidants are essential to your cat's health. My antioxidant formula is in gel form, designed to be given easily. Just let the cat lick the gel or put it on his nose or paws. Formulas are also available in wafer or powdered form.*

DINNER

- 1/4 can professional/alternative diet food

OR

- Just a little less than 1/4 cup dry professional/alternative food with 1 teaspoon professional/alternative canned food
- 1/8 teaspoon SLIM & HEALTHY SUPPLEMENT MIXTURE

BEFORE BED

- Exercise
- Clean teeth
- 1/4 cup chopped veggies
- Optional: popcorn
- Optional: 1/3 cup dry adult or diet food

STRING AND BAG

Some cats love popcorn. They even play with it.

T H U R S D A Y

A.M.

- Just a little less than 1/2 can professional/ alternative diet food

OR

- A scant 1/2 cup dry diet professional/ alternative food with 1 teaspoon professional/ alternative canned food
- 1/8 teaspoon SLIM & HEALTHY SUPPLEMENT MIXTURE
- 1/4 cup chopped veggies
- Optional: a little less than 1/3 cup dry professional/ alternative diet food

We are now cutting down on the canned food (and thus the calories). Your cat will require some canned food in which to hide the supplement.

By now, you should not have trouble giving the Slim & Healthy Supplement Mixture to him, even if you are not at 1/8 teaspoon yet.

Early P.M.

- 1/4 can food with 1/8 teaspoon dandelions or 3–4 drops of tincture

OR

- 1/4 cup dry food with 3/4 teaspoon canned food and 1/8 teaspoon dandelions or 3–4 drops of dandelion tincture
- Comb/groom
- Exercise
- Antioxidant

CLIMB THE MOUNTAIN

The object of this exercise is to burn calories and try to build muscle. Place furniture in such a way that your cat has to climb from the floor, to a love seat, to a sofa back, to a love seat, etc. You may want to use the cord or the fishing pole to entice him. This exercise must be done slowly, especially if your cat is very heavy, that's a lot of weight on those little joints! Three minutes is acceptable—I would like five minutes, but only if your cat is fit!

DINNER

- 1/4 can professional/alternative diet food

OR

- Just a little less than 1/4 cup dry professional/alternative food with 1 teaspoon professional/alternative canned food
- 1/8 teaspoon SLIM & HEALTHY SUPPLEMENT MIXTURE

BEFORE BED

- Clean teeth
- 1/4 cup chopped veggies
- Optional: corn on the cob
- Optional: a little less than 1/3 cup dry diet food

At this point, it may still be hard to brush your cat's teeth. I would like to encourage you to continue. Put water on the toothbrush or finger cot instead of liquid or paste. Let your cat get used to your fingers, or the brush, in his mouth.

You may have the urge to feel for those ribs, but not yet: let's wait until Sunday. Please remember that the amounts of food I have written may not be correct for your brand of food or your cat. Sunday will let you know if you have to decrease the food.

F R I D A Y

A.M.

- Just a little less than 1/2 can professional/ alternative diet food

OR

- Feed a little less than 1/2 cup dry diet professional/ alternative food with 1 teaspoon professional/ alternative canned food
- 1/8 teaspoon SLIM & HEALTHY SUPPLEMENT MIXTURE
- 1/4 cup chopped veggies
- Optional: 1/3 cup dry professional/ alternative diet food

You should be adding the 1/8 teaspoon of the Slim & Healthy Supplement Mixture. You still have more than 3 weeks left on this 30-day diet plan.

Early P.M.

- Fish for Friday:
  Fish Fillet & Garlic
- Comb/groom
- Exercise
- Antioxidant

Fish Fillet & Garlic

White-meat fish (cod, sole)	Sprinkle of parsley
1/8 teaspoon garlic	Pinch of salt
Olive oil	Pinch of fresh or powdered dandelion

Sauté 1/8 teaspoon garlic in enough olive oil to moisten the frying pan. Cook the "white-meat fish" (cod, sole), making sure there are no bones. Sprinkle parsley (fresh is best), add a pinch of salt and serve.

FETCH THE BALL

Take aluminum foil and roll it into a ball the size of a golf ball, or buy foam rubber golf balls. Throw them, and let your cat retrieve them. The more, the better—I would like to see your cat retrieve ten!

Leave some fish for a snack before bedtime.

DINNER

- 1/4 can food with 1/8 teaspoon fresh or powdered dandelion or 3–4 drops of the
  tincture

OR

- 1/4 cup dry diet food + 3/4 teaspoon canned food + 1/8 teaspoon fresh or powdered dandelion or 3–4 drops of the tincture

BEFORE BED

- Exercise
- Clean teeth
- Hair-ball medicine
- 1/4 cup raw or cooked peas (look at the ingredients—no sugar please)
- Left-over fish

FETCH THE BALL

Make balls of various sizes from aluminum foil, or buy foam-rubber balls from the pet store—whatever excites your cat and gets him to move!

comment . . . *By this time, you and your cat are getting used to this routine. If it's still not perfect, that's okay. The important thing is to exercise, and watch the amounts of food being given. You may have to readjust the amounts next week—Sunday will tell.*

S A T U R D A Y

A.M.

- Just a little more than 1/2 can food

OR

- Feed a little less than 1/2 cup dry food with 1/2 teaspoon professional/ alternative canned food
- 1/8 teaspoon SLIM & HEALTHY SUPPLEMENT MIXTURE
- 1/4 cup vegetables or fruit
- Optional: just a little less than 1/3 cup dry professional/ alternative diet food

I have lowered the amount of canned food again. If that is acceptable with your cat, we will continue with that amount for the rest of the diet plan. If you do cut down on food, also reduce the amount of dry food, giving a little less than 1/2 cup.

Let's also decrease the amount of dry food left down.

Early P.M.

- Liver Delight
- Comb/groom
- Exercise
- Antioxidant

Liver Delight

1/2 cup diced liver	1/8 teaspoon minced vegetables
1/8 teaspoon minced garlic	Crushed parsley

Combine liver, garlic and vegetables. Sauté all of it in a small amount of olive oil until done. Add some crushed parsley. Let it cool and serve.

Exercise: Anything you want, make it a little longer than usual, since it's Saturday.

DINNER
- 1/3 can professional/alternative diet food

OR
- Just a little less than 1/4 cup dry professional/alternative food with 1 teaspoon professional/alternative canned food
- 1/8 teaspoon SLIM & HEALTHY SUPPLEMENT MIXTURE

BEFORE BED	Any exercise you want.

BEFORE BED
- Exercise
- Clean teeth
- 1/4 cup chopped vegetables
- Optional: less than 1/3 cup dry diet food
- Optional: corn on the cob

comment . . . *Don't forget to grow wheat grass in a small flower pot for your cat. The fiber is good for him.*

S U N D A Y

A.M.
- Just a little more than 1/3 can food

OR
- Feed even less than 1/2 cup dry food with 1/2 teaspoon professional/ alternative canned food
- 1/8 teaspoon Slim & Healthy Supplement Mixture
- 1/4 cup chopped veggies
- NO DRY FOOD

NO DRY FOOD. If you absolutely have to, give him 10 nuggets.

***comment* . . .** *You should be giving your cat the full measure of 1/8 teaspoon of the Slim & Healthy Supplement Mixture.*

Early P.M.

- Fish Fillet & Garlic
- Comb/groom
- Exercise
- Antioxidant

Fish Fillet & Garlic

- White-meat fish (cod, sole)
- 1/8 teaspoon garlic
- Olive oil
- Sprinkle of parsley
- Pinch of salt
- Pinch of fresh or powdered dandelion

Sauté 1/8 teaspoon garlic in enough olive oil to moisten the frying pan. Cook the "white-meat fish" (cod, sole), making sure there are no bones. Sprinkle parsley (fresh is best), add a pinch of salt and serve.

The amount of food you give the cat will have to be adjusted, depending on your cat's weight loss, if any. Remember, fast weight loss is not healthy. Your cat should lose no more than 1/2 pound per week.

DINNER

- 1/3 can professional/alternative diet food

OR

- Just a little less than 1/4 cup dry professional/alternative food with 1 teaspoon professional/alternative canned food
- 1/8 teaspoon SLIM & HEALTHY SUPPLEMENT MIXTURE

BEFORE BED

- Exercise
- Clean teeth
- 1/4 cup chopped vegetables
- Optional: less than 1/3 cup dry diet food
- Optional: corn on the cob

Try cucumbers if you still haven't found a vegetable your cat likes.

If your cat just refuses vegetables, try puffed rice cereal (dry). If that fails, you will have to use dry diet food, but eventually no more than 10–20 nuggets!

Now it's time for the weekly examination. Weigh yourself on a scale. Hold your cat and weigh yourself again. Subtract your weight without the cat, from your weight with the cat. That will tell you how much your cat weighs. Record the exam and the weight. If your cat did not lose weight, reduce the food by 10%. If your cat did lose 1/4–1/2 lb., that's perfect; continue the same amount as last week. Your goal for next week is 1/2 pound less.

comment . . . *This week will be much easier for you. You will know how much food to feed, and how much of the supplements to add. If you are still not sure about it, you will have it down by the middle of the week. Wait until you see how good your cat is going to look and feel!*

After the 30-day plan, you may follow the adult or geriatric plan, or if you want, you may continue this plan.

Weekly examination

Place your cat on the table as you would to clean its teeth and gums. Mark your rating 1 to 3 in the box below. Go back to the questions for the weekly examination on pages 208-210.

PHYSICAL APPEARANCE	WEEK 1	WEEK 2	WEEK 3	WEEK 4
Looking at your cat from a distance:				
waist line	☐	☐	☐	☐
stomach	☐	☐	☐	☐
Looking at your cat close up:				
whiskers	☐	☐	☐	☐
eyes	☐	☐	☐	☐
breath	☐	☐	☐	☐
coat	☐	☐	☐	☐
skin	☐	☐	☐	☐
tail	☐	☐	☐	☐
nails & pads	☐	☐	☐	☐
ribs	☐	☐	☐	☐
BODILY FUNCTIONS				
appetite	☐	☐	☐	☐
hair balls	☐	☐	☐	☐
stool	☐	☐	☐	☐
BEHAVIOR				
activity	☐	☐	☐	☐

CHAPTER 11

Special Problems, Special Diets

Allergies

*Allergic reactions vary from cat to cat,
frequently causing confusion.*

Some cats are allergic, while others are sensitive to something. Allergic or sensitive, the symptoms exist. Studies show that only a very small number of cats are actually allergic, even though *we* say they are allergic.

An allergy is a specific type of cellular reaction to a substance called an allergen, which is generally a protein. A sensitivity is also a reaction to a substance, but on a different chemical level. That substance can be a protein as well as other things, such as dyes and preservatives. The type of reaction a cat has when some substance is bothering him varies from cat to cat, depending on age, physical condition, amount of contact with the substance, and the severity of the reaction.

For the purpose of this section, I will use the term allergic, but I am including sensitivity reactions as well.

Reaction possibilities

Diarrhea, vomiting, skin lesions, hives, runny eyes, coughing, sneezing, itching, scratching, swelling, dermatitis, hair loss, and more. The truth is: most food-allergic cats show skin disease, rather than gastrointestinal problems. Food sensitivity can manifest as vomiting, runny eyes, etc.

Contact possibilities

- Ingestion (of certain foods, herbs, medications)
- Inhalation (of pollens, smoke, dust, powders, polishes, feathers, mold)
- Interaction (with certain types of material, dyes, flea collars, powders, soaps, carpets, grass)
- Injection (of insect venom [stings], medications)

Don't jump to conclusions

Before assuming your cat's symptoms are allergic reactions, I'd suggest having your pet checked by a veterinarian to eliminate the possibility of disease or infection. The next step is to discover the offending substance; the best way is by process of elimination.

Allergen elimination diet

To pinpoint a food allergen or a sensitive food substance, a diet composed of ingredients that the cat hasn't eaten recently or frequently and are known for producing an allergic response must be fed exclusively for two weeks. Absolutely no other foods should be given. Only distilled water is allowed for the first two weeks; tap water is recommended as the first dietary addition. Keep in mind that the recipe is not 100% nutritional, but for two weeks, it will not harm your cat.

> 4 ounces boiled rabbit, venison or lamb
> 1 cup long-grain, cooked white rice, no instant rice

There are commercial venison, lamb and rabbit diets for cats available. The problem is that some contain vitamins, minerals, and brewer's yeast—and are, therefore, not TRULY just lamb, venison or rabbit. If you absolutely can't prepare the above recipe, then by all means try one of the commercial brands from your veterinarian.

If your cat shows improvement after two weeks on this regimen, you may begin adding new foods to the diet, but at the rate of only one ingredient a week. This way, if there's no recurrence of allergic symptoms, you'll know the new food is okay for permanent use in the diet. Begin by adding proteins (beef, liver, poultry, fish, eggs, milk), and then introduce cereal and grain products (oatmeal, cornmeal, barley). Once this is done, find a quality canned or dry food that contains only the ingredients well-tolerated by your cat.

If no improvement is shown during the two weeks of the regimen, your cat's problem may not be a food allergy, and other possibilities should be investigated; I'd recommend consulting your veterinarian. Keep in mind that anything can cause a reaction: a hair-ball remedy, a vitamin tablet, a food additive, a cookie, a flea bite—items so seemingly inconsequential that you might never have even considered them. What's important to remember about allergies, and sensitivities, is that little things do mean a lot and can do a lot of mean things, especially to susceptible cats.

True, allergic reactions are generally limited to protein substances, but, as I've said, for the cat owner allergy *vs.* sensitivity is meaningless. One or more offending substances have to be eliminated in any case.

Anorexia

How to give your cat more than a slim chance at renewed health

Refusal of food for more than two days is abnormal feline behavior. Loss of appetite (anorexia) in cats is always potentially life-threatening and must never be ignored. With this disease, once your pet stops eating, he no longer wants to eat, then won't eat, and eventually, can't eat. Whether the cause is emotional (fright, hostility, depression), brought on by a new environment or pet, or physical (pain, injury, trauma), brought on by oral dysfunction, internal obstruction, or illness, the results can be disastrous without quick action, and the right nourishment.

Quick action for anorexia

Bring your cat to a veterinarian as soon as possible. An anorectic cat should not be confused with a finicky eater.

The right nourishment for an anorectic cat

- Water is the most important nutrient and is required in large amounts. Cats will instinctively cut back on food and physical activity to decrease water loss.
- Increase caloric intake by adding honey to the water. Although physically inactive, your cat's caloric needs will usually increase in proportion to the severity of the disease or condition, responsible for the anorexia.
- Increase protein supply. Protein needs are greater in anorectic cats and must be met with easily digested, and utilized, high-BV quality sources. Egg yolks or soft-boiled eggs are easy to feed.
- Lactose-free milk, plus honey and an egg yolk, adds up to fair nourishment.
- Provide vitamin and mineral dietary supplements. In the cat's debilitated condition, daily pediatric doses of zinc, vitamin B complex, and vitamin C, are recommended.
- Give plenty of stroking and loving. This helps food go down and keeps your cat's spirits up.

Restarting stalled appetites

- Mix one ounce of water with two to four ounces of a high-fat, easily digestible, calorie-dense (and tasty) professional food, such as canned Prescription Diet Feline P/D (Hill's), or add water to IAMS kitten food, forming a semi-liquid consistency.
- Feed small amounts four to six times daily.
- Finger-feed (as opposed to force-feed) your cat by placing pill-size portions of food on his tongue.
- Offer baby-food chicken and rice. This is intended *only* as a temporary, fast-fix appetite stimulant. After a day or two, the cat should be eased onto a complete, nutritionally balanced diet. Gradually replace small portions of the baby food with a

quality alternative food. Heating (not cooking) the meal will enhance flavor.

Arthritis

Cats with a difficult joint problem

This painful joint condition is a common affliction of aging cats. Their hindquarters become stiff; movement is difficult; sometimes, even waking up, seems hard for them. Cortisone drugs relieve pain, but I feel that unless drugs are absolutely necessary, a cat is better off without them.

Comfort and nutrition count

- Keep the cat in a warm area, away from dampness and drafts.
- Make the litter box easily accessible.
- Feed a quality professional/alternative food with high-BV protein and maximum digestibility. Count those calories, however—a fat cat puts more weight on his bones.
- Supplement the daily diet with the following:

  1/8 teaspoon ACA
  (an alfalfa supplement by
  Natural Animal, 1-800-548-2899)
  and/or
  Alfalfa tincture as per directions from Animals'
  Apawthecary (1-800-822-9609)
  and/or

  GlycoFlex—veterinarian RX needed
  Vetri Science Laboratories
  Essex Junction, Vermont
  and
  Omega 3 and Omega 6 oil supplement (Gold
  Caps, Dr. Jane® Essential Gold, Derm Caps,
  Opticoat II)
  and
  Antioxidant Formula

Cancer

Not all types are curable, but some may be preventable, and may make cancer therapy more tolerable.

By definition, cancer is a malignant tumor that invades other tissue by moving from one part of the body to another, growing on (and destroying) healthy cells.

Preventive feeding

There is no cure-all diet for cancer, but a cat with a strong immune system is certainly far better equipped to withstand the rigors of treatment, less likely to succumb to infection during recuperation, and most likely able to spend many more happy years with you.

Recommended foods and supplements

NOTE: If your cat is being treated for cancer or any other illness, do not make any dietary changes or supplement additions without first consulting your veterinarian.

- Quality professional/alternative canned and dry food containing high-BV protein, fat, and numerous vitamins and minerals, with as few carbohydrates as possible
- 250–500 mg of vitamin C daily, or an antioxidant formula
- 50–100 IU vitamin E daily, or an antioxidant formula
- Omega 3 fat supplement daily. (Follow manufacturer's recommendation.) Dr. Jane® Essential Gold, Derm Caps, are examples.
- Acidophilus: two tablespoons plain yogurt or one squeeze Bene Bac, manufactured by Pet Ag
- 1/4 teaspoon brewer's or torula yeast and bran mix added to food once a day
- Shark Cartilage—follow appropriate dose
- Nothing that contains sodium nitrite or artificial coloring

No food or supplement regimen is a guarantee against illness, but my New-Life Nutrition Plan in chapter 10 can offer your cat the best possible chance at good health.

Diabetes

Top dietary management is required at all feeding levels.

When a cat's pancreas fails to produce adequate insulin, the hormone necessary for proper metabolism and maintenance levels of blood sugar (glucose), the result is an improper metabolism of carbohydrates, an uncontrolled rise in blood sugar, and a disease called Diabetes Mellitus.

In cats, increased thirst and increased urine production are usually symptoms owners notice first, and thankfully, rarely ignore. Once a diagnosis is made and these cats are put on medication, a strict diabetes management diet, or both, they can live long, happy, active lives.

There are various natural compounds which can effectively manage diabetes. They must be prescribed by a veterinarian since they can radically decrease your cat's insulin needs. Call the American Holistic Veterinary Association (410-569-0795) to find a veterinarian in your area.

Firm feeding rules for your diabetic cat

1. In order to establish and maintain a correct insulin dosage, you must feed the same amount of food with the same ingredients every day. A fixed-formula food with quality protein, quality-controlled processing, high palatability, and a low carbohydrate content, is not an option—it's a necessity.
2. Supermarket foods are generally not fixed formulas, so a professional/alternative food is necessary. Adding fiber will help regulate your cat. Try 1/8 teaspoon of oat bran mixed with 1/8 teaspoon of brewer's or torula yeast—start with a pinch, until you can work up to 1/4 teaspoon daily, or feed a high-fiber food as recommended by your veternarian.
3. Never make any dietary changes or additions without consulting your veterinarian. Although a diet with more fiber may be healthy for your cat (and high-fiber diets are), a switch could necessitate a reduction of the animal's prescribed insulin dosage—and that's a decision only your pet's doctor is qualified to make.
4. Feed your cat twice daily, but only high-protein, low-carbohydrate, meals.

5. Don't let your cat get fat. If his current food is making him fat—
   adjust the amount. If he still continues to gain, then a diet food is
   necessary.
6. The cat's diet should be supplemented with 100–300 mg vitamin C
   or an antioxidant formula.

Fleas

A flea can be a lot more than a little pest. These are hardy villains
and can live for up to two years in your home. They can cause allergies, parasite infections, skin conditions and more. They should be
kept out of your home and off your pet. Ask your veterinarian for a
safe and effective cure.

Feeding for protection

Though no studies prove it, I've seen cats on brewer's or torula
yeast and garlic with fewer fleas than before they were on it. The
yeast and garlic also keep the skin healthy so that when your cat
scratches, it causes less damage to the skin. If you can't find a mixture of torula or brewer's yeast and garlic, add fresh or canned garlic
to the food along with the yeast. Powdered garlic is not an acceptable alternative.

Feline Leukemia (FeLV)

*Some cats are carriers, others are victims, but all are
potential targets for this cancerous virus.*

Highly contagious, this feline viral blood cancer is spread through
the saliva (possibly also the urine and feces) of infected cats. Once the
disease is contracted, a cat generally does not survive for more than a
few years, despite medical treatment.

The symptoms include: jaundice, anemia, weight loss, appetite
loss, diarrhea or constipation, enlarged lymph nodes, fatigue, excessive thirst and/or urination, respiratory distress, infertility, and probably a deteriorating immune system that prevents victims from

warding off other diseases. As yet, there is no cure, but vaccines are available. Ask your veterinarian about testing for feline leukemia and vaccine options.

Feeding for fortification

A healthy adult cat, exposed to the virus, can develop immunity to the primary disease (in effect, suppress it), and live out a normal life. But should this carrier's natural defenses be nutritionally let down, particularly during a period of stress, the disease could then surface and strike.

Recipe for resistance

- Vary feeding of professional/alternative canned and dry foods that contain high-BV protein in a good ratio to quality fat, with an impressive vitamin-mineral analysis, add no artificial coloring or sodium nitrite, and no more than one preservative.
- Provide 1/4 teaspoon of bee pollen or Dr. Jane® Beezyme daily.
- 250–500 mg of vitamin C daily.
- Provide an antioxidant formula daily.
- Provide balanced Omega 3/6 fatty-acid supplement with zinc daily.
- Shark cartilage.

FLUTD (Feline Lower Urologic Syndrome)

Feline Lower Urologic Syndrome (FLUTD) is one of the most common and painful cat ailments, sending thousands of cats a year to veterinary hospitals and probably an equal number of owners up the wall. Ironically, it's one of the most preventable feline problems.

Characterized by frequent, strained voiding of small quantities of odorous, often bloody, urine in locations other than the litter box, FLUTD is essentially caused by the presence of calculi in the urinary tract, where they can promote obstruction, serious urethral irritation, and dangerous blockage.

Avoiding and treating FLUTD

- Feed a food that produces an acidic urine.
- Feed a diet low in magnesium and high in calories. The greater a food's caloric density, the less a cat needs to consume. Decrease magnesium intake, and thereby its presence in the urine.
- Keep the litter box clean and provide fresh water daily. No hard water, please. It usually contains too much magnesium for a cat's comfort.
- Free feed. This keeps the urine at the most consistant pH.
- Be wary of supermarket/commercial "low ash" foods. Ash is the residue of many minerals your cat needs. What you want to know is the level of magnesium in that ash, which your cat doesn't need. For prevention of calculi formation, you want foods to contain less than .1% dry matter basis, or about .02% of wet food.
- Feed only foods with high-BV protein (meat, poultry, fish, eggs) that usually produce acidic urine. Other proteins, such as soybean meal, wheat middlings, corn gluten meal, and so on, generally do not produce acidic urine, and they rank pretty low on my nutritional scale, too.
- Encourage increased liquid intake. Sneak a tablespoon or two of water, broth or tomato juice into all canned meals. If necessary, and sodium is not restricted, you can probably get your cat to drink without having to lead it to water, by adding a pinch of salt to its food.
- Avoid high-magnesium treats, such as shrimp, sardines or nuts, and feed only foods that are acceptable for FLUTD management.
- Don't add brewer's yeast (0.17 percent magnesium) to food if your cat has a FLUTD problem.
- Beware of food with many cereals that produce an acidic urine. Too much acid is dangerous and it's often added to change the urine pH. The pH should not be less than 6.0. Call the manufacturer and ask what the urine pH is: they must supply you with that information.
- Give your cat chloreito (an herb), it's known to decrease stru-

vite crystal formation. Since dosage varies with the product, give 1/10 the adult dosage recommended on the package.

Heart Disease

Where the heart is concerned, a cat is never too old or too young to have problems.

Cardiovascular ailments can afflict cats of all ages. Although there is a wide variety of heart problems, differing in severity and symptoms (which range from simple weakness, mild coughing, weight loss, labored breathing, abdominal distension and collapse), all are cause for concern and treatment.

The proper functioning of a cat's vital organs depends on the health of the cardiovascular system. In order to retain and restore his health, dietary management is essential.

Pass on the salt

Reducing the cat's intake of sodium is of primary importance, since salt causes water retention. Water retention puts a heavier load on kidneys, already overworked and under-fueled because of impaired cardiac function, and can result in heart failure.

Knowing the right "No's" for the heart

- No smoked foods, or any luncheon meats. Also, avoid shellfish, canned soups, foods with monosodium glutamate (MSG, Accent), processed cheeses, breads and cereals, canned vegetables, and people food in general.
- No cat foods that list salt as an ingredient. (Commercial cat food ingredients already contain salt, so an additional listing means there's much more in there than your cat can handle safely.)
- No protein other than that of the highest utilizable quality. You don't want any more waste material going through the kidneys than necessary, and you do want your pet to get the best amino acids possible.
- No water treated by a home water softener. Home water softeners add sodium. If you are unsure about the sodium content

of your tap water, provide distilled water and encourage your pet to drink.

- No added supplements if you are feeding your pet a prescription diet, such as Feline H/D, CV-Formula Feline Diet. Prescription diets are carefully formulated, and supplement additions, with the exception of brewer's or torula yeast (which is advised because of its B vitamins and anti-stress properties), and vegetable enzymes, can undermine the nutrient ratio designed to maintain a correct electrolyte balance.
- There are some beneficial effects from various herbs and natural compounds but these require a veterinarian's prescription.

A few heart-to-heart tips and cautions

- If your cat is overweight, decrease portion sizes of his low-salt meals. Unless specifically prescribed, avoid feeding prepared reducing diets, since they are usually high in salt.
- Chopped cucumbers and dandelions are natural diuretics, which increase urine excretion, and can be added to food.
- Supplement the cat's diet with a balanced vitamin B complex (or brewer's or torula yeast), and vitamin C daily, and 50–100 IU of vitamin E, daily. Ask your veterinarian first, however.
- If you are preparing homemade meals, do not use baking soda as an ingredient.
- Exercise is important, but consult your vet on how much your cat is allowed.

Dr. Jane's Sans-Salt Supper

The following recipe should interest the most finicky cat. Since it's not 100% balanced, it's meant only as an occasional treat—no more than 2–3 times weekly.

Kidney Disease

Not all old cats have it, and many young cats do.

One of the most widely propagated health myths about cats is that if they're old and they're sick, they have kidney disease. And

Dr. Jane's Sans-Salt Supper

4 oz. cooked ground beef	1/4 teaspoon calcium carbonate or other calcium supplement without sodium (available at health food stores and pharmacies)
1 oz. cooked beef liver	
1/4 cup cooked (without salt) long-grain white rice (not "instant" rice)	
1/4 teaspoon corn oil	1/4 teaspoon brewer's yeast or torula yeast
	1 thin slice cucumber, finely chopped

Braise beef and liver in small amount of unsalted water in a covered saucepan. Cook 5–10 minutes, depending upon whether your cat prefers meat rare, medium, or well done. Chop liver into tiny chunks. Transfer cooked beef and liver to feeding dish and mix in remaining ingredients. Add as much cooking liquid as needed to achieve desired consistency. Test food to see that it's cooled to room temperature before serving.

this just isn't true! Granted, as cats age, there is a gradual, natural deceleration of kidney function, but this is not kidney disease! And considering the abundance of inferior protein being foisted on cats these days, it's remarkable that it isn't.

The kidneys, which are responsible for gathering and distributing needed nutrients and eliminating harmful substances from the blood, spend most of their time excreting waste from nutrient breakdown. This means that the less quality a protein has, the more work the kidneys must do. Conversely, more quality protein means less work for the kidneys.

Owner alert

Kidney disease symptoms (scratching, mangy coat, fatigue, increased thirst, frequent urination), indicative as they might appear, are not proof of the disease. Without a BUN (blood, urea, nitrogen concentration) test and urine test to determine the levels at which the kidneys are functioning, no accurate diagnosis can be made.

Because the disease can strike cats of all ages, I recommend that your pet be given a BUN and other tests annually after the age of six. The earlier potential problems are detected, the easier the disease is to prevent.

Prevention is as easy as 1-2-3

1. Switch your pet to a high-BV protein professional/alternative food and serve it twice daily.
2. If the cat is overweight, it's instant shape-up time.
3. Supplement his diet with:
     1/4 teaspoon torula yeast twice daily with food
     1/4 teaspoon crushed garlic (contains potassium)
     plenty of fresh water daily

What to do if your cat has kidney problems

If a BUN and other tests show that your cat has a kidney disease, or renal damage that has impaired proper kidney function, you must pay strict attention to special nutritional guidelines.

- Protein intake must be moderated and limited to highest quality sources; the extent of protein limitation is determined by how effectively, and at what level, the kidneys are functioning. (At one time, it was recommended to restrict protein during kidney disease, but I suggest that it is necessary to limit protein only when kidney function is very poor.)
- Sodium intake must be restricted. (See suggestions in "Heart Disease" section.)
- Phosphorus intake must be restricted. Avoid foods with an inverse calcium/phosphorus ratio.
- Provide professional, fixed-formula food with restricted high-quality protein and minerals, such as Prescription Diet Feline K/D.
- Add crushed garlic to make up for potassium loss.
- Supplement his diet with B vitamins.
- Plenty of fresh water.

There are many herbal and natural compounds which may be helpful to your cat but should be administered only by a veterinarian. To locate an appropriate vet in your area, contact the American Holistic Veterinary Association (410-569-0795).

Liver (Hepatic) Disease

*Even a cat with nine lives has only one liver, and
it's vital that you know how to care for it.*

The liver is your pet's frontline fighter against invading poisons,
pathogens and toxins; the engineer in charge of storing and effi-
ciently dispensing fat, fat-soluble vitamins, and glycogen; the
provider of blood-clotting vitamin K; the force behind effective carbohydrate, fat and protein metabolism, bile production, and more.
Needless to say, when this organ becomes diseased, your cat's life depends on its recovery.

Multiple symptoms and causes

Lethargy, weight loss, anemia, jaundice, diarrhea and vomiting
are only a few of the numerous distress signals indicating liver trouble. Liver trouble can stem from an equally large number of causes,
and is, therefore, one of the few diseases more difficult to prevent
than to treat, which is why understanding the management of this
ailment is so important.

Get-well notes to remember

1. Feed your pet restricted amounts of thoroughly digestible, utilizable, high-BV protein, but not a high-protein diet. This might
   sound contradictory, but it's not. The point is to reduce the liver's
   work load, which involves removal of waste from amino acids,
   and to provide relief for the kidneys, while still supplying quality
   protein needed for recovery.
2. If your pet has no appetite, follow the advice given in the section
   on anorexia, but do not feed baby food. Baby food hasn't enough
   of the necessary balanced protein, fat, minerals, and vitamins,
   and often has too much phosphorus. Prescription Diet Feline
   K/D (Hill's) is properly formulated for liver ailments and can be
   made into a liquid preparation by adding distilled water.
3. Salt and phosphorus intake should be restricted. (More relief for
   the kidneys, which have no choice but to be involved when
   there's liver trouble.)

4. Equal parts of cottage cheese and cooked brown rice are highly digestible and work well as a diet in the early stages of the illness. A soft-boiled egg (or raw egg yolk) mixed in adds palatability. This should not be used as an extended, long-term diet, since it doesn't contain the proper balance of necessary vitamins and minerals, but it can be added anytime to a prescription diet that needs a flavor booster.

5. Add no additional fats to food, and give no fat-soluble vitamins. (Again, too much work for the liver.)

6. Keep methionine and choline out of the diet. The intestines will convert these into mercaptans, which are toxic, and with the liver unable to oust them from the body, encephalopathy, a dysfunctioning of the brain, can occur.

7. Feed small amounts of food four to six times daily. This gives the debilitated liver a chance to relax between work loads.

8. B vitamins, with the exception of choline, are recommended as daily supplements. The Bs are stress fighters. Be sure they're given together in equal dosage. Too much of one can deplete the others.

9. Restrict foods with fish meal, melts (spleens of slaughtered animals), and other glandular products (shellfish and meats). The liver is in no condition to handle their wastes, which can cause an unwanted buildup of uric acid.

10. When adding carbohydrates to the diet, use easily digestible buckwheat groats (kasha), oatmeal or cornmeal (polenta). Only add carbohydrates if your cat is getting enough protein. Do not use whole corn, which is hard to digest.

11. 50–100 mg of vitamin C daily.

12. 10 mg zinc every other day.

Obesity

*With the exception of Garfield, it's no fun
for a cat to be fat.*

Some cats are naturally round and puffy-looking; others are naturally lean and muscular (see chapter 6 for descriptions of different breeds). But no cat is naturally fat.

You should suspect that your cat is overweight if his abdomen and/or chest sags; if he has difficulty grooming himself; if you try to feel his rib cage and can't.

You should know that your cat is overweight if you say, "Here, kitty, kitty," and then feel the house shake, can't see his paws, or find he needs a forklift to get into the litter box. If you don't realize this, you're both in BIG trouble.

A cat that's overweight can develop serious problems. Once excess pounds pile on, normal exercise and movement slack off, along with daily hygiene. Twisting his body to wash the hindquarters or genital area becomes increasingly difficult, and eventually, the animal gives up. Before long, the result of neglect becomes visible: dull hair becomes matted and sparse, and small lesions provide moist havens for bacteria, turning minor skin irritations into persistent infections. And this is only the beginning.

Weighty problems for overweight cats

No matter what the disease (kidney, heart, lung, etc.), excessive weight worsens it.

Diabetes
The more a cat eats, the higher his blood sugar, the more insulin he needs, and the harder his pancreas has to work. Without a change of pace—or diet—insulin cells could burn out and diabetes could set in.

Heart and liver diseases
Fat doesn't accumulate only in visible areas, but also around the heart and liver. The former decreases blood flow to organs, and causes numerous cardiovascular as well as respiratory problems; the latter creates serious digestive disorders and a conglomeration of interrelated illnesses.

Decreased resistance to infection
Extra weight overworks all vital organs, stresses the body, depletes nutrients, weakens the immune system, and prevents efficient production of protective antibodies.

Ounce-for-ounce, pound-for-pound prevention

Feline obesity occurs when a cat's calorie intake exceeds his bodily needs and daily energy expenditure. This could be caused by hypothyroidism, which slows down the metabolism rate at which calories are normally consumed, but it's usually caused by obesity, which is a preventable disease, and it's up to you to prevent it!

- Determine what your cat should weigh, then feed him only enough calories to maintain that weight.
- Don't get in the habit of creating bad habits, such as giving between meal snacks; offering food from the table just because you happen to be eating at the moment, and your pet isn't; using food as a reward; or providing an assortment of meals for your finicky eater (who'll end up eating more than a fair share of all of them).
- Know the approximate calories of foods you feed and avoid those high in carbohydrates and sugar.
- Substitute vegetables for high-calorie commercial snacks.
- Don't leave food down for more than twenty minutes. A cat who's allowed to eat whenever he wants, will get into the habit of eating more often—and more than he should.
- Divide his meal into multiples. The more often a cat eats, the more weight it loses and is less prone to FLUTD. Be careful not to feed more in six meals than you would in 2–3 meals.
- Don't use milk as a substitute for water.
- Play with your pet often. A cat kept on his paws is easier to keep in shape.
- Don't keep your house too warm. It tends to make cats lazy, less active, and larger.
- If your cat is a competitive eater, feed away from other animals, or at another time.
- Use your eyes and your head when feeding. If your cat looks as if he's gaining weight, cut back on the portion size. It's as simple as that. Unless you've let things go too far and have to put your cat on a real diet, just reduce the amount of food gradually. That's only fair. After all, you're the one who should have been counting the calories.

When it's time to diet

If your cat is overweight and you must put him on a diet, my advice is to get on Dr. Jane's 30-Day Obesity Diet and/or get a professional reducing food, such as Prescription Diet Feline R/D (Hill's) or OM-Formula Feline Diet (Purina). It's high in fiber and provides enough bulk to satisfy a cat that's used to eating a substantial quantity of food. Once your cat has lost the extra weight, Iams Less Active Cat Food will maintain it. I don't encourage long-term use of high fibers.

If you're restricting your pet's total food intake, remember that it means you're restricting intake of necessary vitamins and minerals, too. A balanced supplement must be given daily. I'd suggest Dr. Jane® Beezyme or bee pollen and vegetable enzymes, and adding crushed dandelions to your cat's food. This will help with weight reduction.

Worms (Intestinal Parasites)

Once they're in your cat, they can take a lot out of him.

If your cat spends time outdoors and is the sort unlikely to pass up any recreational eating that's within paw's reach, chances are he has worms. By no means does this imply that you're to rush out for medicine and immediately worm your pet. In fact, I strongly caution against doing so.

No worm medication should ever be given to a cat before a diagnosis has been made by a veterinarian, especially since the general symptoms of parasite infestation (vomiting, diarrhea, grass eating, fatigue, dull coat, running eyes, weight loss) could be indicators of numerous diseases. Furthermore, over-the-counter worm medication can be extremely harmful to many cats. If improperly administered, or given under the wrong circumstances, it could be lethal. Never worm a kitten or a cat who's pregnant, nursing, sick, or geriatric without professional supervision.

The most common intestinal parasites are roundworms, hookworms, tapeworms and whipworms. Roundworms are frequently passed from an infected queen to her kittens. Tapeworms are usually contracted by cats who have eaten fleas. *Taxoplasmosis gondii* is a parasite that can be found in cats and passed to humans. Immune-compromised people are susceptible to this parasite. Pregnant women tend to worry about it, but in reality, the chance of your cat passing these eggs, and being infectious at the same time, is really very slim. If your pediatrician suggests you get rid of your cat because there is a CHANCE of this parasite, talk to your veterinarian and get information to the doctor ASAP. There is more chance of a pregnant woman getting this disease from planting the garden, than loving her cat. I do, however, advise pregnant women not to change the litter boxes.

Nutrition is your cat's best protection

- Feed the optimal New-Life Diet.
- Supplement all meals with 1/4 teaspoon of brewer's yeast (unless your pet has a FLUTD problem).
- Give 100–200 mg of vitamin C daily.
- Give 1/8–1/4 teaspoon of fresh garlic daily.
- Probiotics are a must (Bene Bac by Pet Ag or Florazyme). Powdered probiotics given in an infant's dose is another choice.

If your cat has worms

- Take it to your veterinarian.
- Feed a professional/alternative food. If your cat has tapeworms and can't keep weight on, feed kitten food because of its extra calories.
- Feed as often as you can—leaving dry down to nibble on.
- Add brewer's or torula yeast and garlic to each meal.

Q&A

Nonessentials About Neutering

Will neutering my cats make them more vulnerable to obesity and FLUTD?

Neutering a cat, male or female, will generally cause a decrease in physical activity, which can predispose the cat to obesity and FLUTD if dietary precautions are not taken. But if you take these precautions and encourage exercise, a neutered cat is no more vulnerable than one who is not neutered.

Allergy vs. Intolerance

My cat has been diagnosed as having a milk intolerance. Is there any difference between an intolerance and an allergy? And if so, what is it?

Yes, there is a difference. Diarrhea is the most common adverse reaction in adult cats. This is due to an intolerance of the lactose (milk sugar) in milk, caused by an insufficiency of the digestive enzyme lactase. A milk allergy, on the other hand, is a hypersensitivity to the protein in milk and can cause other allergic symptoms.

With a lactose intolerance, your cat is usually still able to eat cheese and butter, with no ill effects. With a milk allergy, all forms have to be eliminated from the diet. Any cat food containing whey or casein, for example, cannot be fed. I should add that it's not uncommon for cats allergic to milk to also react adversely to beef.

The Itch-Scratch-Itch Syndrome

I've been told that my cat, Murray (an eight-year-old, neutered male shorthair), has neurological dermatitis. I don't quite understand what this is and why it keeps recurring. I'd greatly appreciate a simple explanation, and any suggestions you might have for treatment.

I wish there were a simple explanation, but because every cat is an individual, there isn't. Neurological dermatitis is a condition in which an animal licks, scratches or bites himself in a specific region for no apparent reason. This usually results in a secondary infection, which causes more itching and scratching, subsequently establishing a vicious cycle.

There are cortisone drugs that can alleviate itching, but cats, being creatures of habit, often resume this self-destructive behavior, possibly when under stress, or if subjected to whatever irritant might have initiated the condition, thereby restarting the cycle. Omega 3/6 fat supplements, Dr. Jane® Essential Gold, Derm Caps, Gold Caps, or

Lipiderm, usually decrease the itching. Antihistamines, such as Chlor-Trimeton, are helpful, but should only be given under veterinary advice.

Fortifying Murray with brewer's or torula yeast and a combination of vitamins C, A, and E, and zinc (a good antioxidant formula should contain this), along with a high-BV-protein, quality-fat diet, will help. Bee pollen or Dr. Jane® Beezyme can also be useful.

Behavior probably plays a role in this disease. Spend lots of TLC time at scheduled intervals, so your cat can count on it. If you think anxiety has a role in this, add chamomile tea to Murray's meals, and Bach Rescue Remedy to the water.

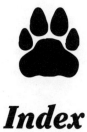

Index

· ·